Psychiatric Emergencies

What Do I Do Now?: Emergency Medicine

SERIES EDITORS-IN-CHIEF

Catherine A. Marco, MD, FACEP
Professor, Emergency Medicine & Surgery
Wright State University Boonshoft School of Medicine
Dayton, Ohio

OTHER VOLUMES IN THE SERIES

Psychiatric Emergencies

Edited by Eileen F. Baker

Emergency Physician, Riverwood Emergency Services, Perrysburg, OH, USA

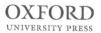

OXFORD
UNIVERSITY PRESS

OXFORD
UNIVERSITY PRESS

Oxford University Press is a department of the University of Oxford. It furthers
the University's objective of excellence in research, scholarship, and education
by publishing worldwide. Oxford is a registered trade mark of Oxford University
Press in the UK and certain other countries.

Published in the United States of America by Oxford University Press
198 Madison Avenue, New York, NY 10016, United States of America.

Library of Congress Cataloging-in-Publication Data
Names: Baker, Eileen F. author.
Title: Psychiatric emergencies / Edited by Eileen F. Baker.
Other titles: What do I do now?
Description: New York, NY : Oxford University Press, [2022] |
Series: What do i do now?: emergency medicine |
Includes bibliographical references and index.
Identifiers: LCCN 2021034901 (print) | LCCN 2021034902 (ebook) |
ISBN 9780197544464 (paperback) | ISBN 9780197544488 (epub) |
ISBN 9780197544495 (online)
Subjects: MESH: Emergency Services, Psychiatric | Crisis Intervention |
Case Reports
Classification: LCC RC439 (print) | LCC RC439 (ebook) | NLM WM 401 |
DDC 362.2/1—dc23
LC record available at https://lccn.loc.gov/2021034901
LC ebook record available at https://lccn.loc.gov/2021034902

DOI: 10.1093/med/9780197544464.001.0001

This material is not intended to be, and should not be considered, a substitute for medical or other
professional advice. Treatment for the conditions described in this material is highly dependent on
the individual circumstances. And, while this material is designed to offer accurate information with
respect to the subject matter covered and to be current as of the time it was written, research and
knowledge about medical and health issues is constantly evolving and dose schedules for medications
are being revised continually, with new side effects recognized and accounted for regularly. Readers
must therefore always check the product information and clinical procedures with the most up-to-date
published product information and data sheets provided by the manufacturers and the most recent
codes of conduct and safety regulation. The publisher and the authors make no representations or
warranties to readers, express or implied, as to the accuracy or completeness of this material. Without
limiting the foregoing, the publisher and the authors make no representations or warranties as to the
accuracy or efficacy of the drug dosages mentioned in the material. The authors and the publisher do
not accept, and expressly disclaim, any responsibility for any liability, loss, or risk that may be claimed
or incurred as a consequence of the use and/or application of any of the contents of this material.

9 8 7 6 5 4 3 2 1
Printed by Marquis, Canada

Contents

Contributors

Mara S. Aloi, MD
Department of Emergency
    Medicine
Allegheny General Hospital
Pittsburgh, PA, USA

Bryan Balentine, MD
Assistant System Medical Director
Department of Emergency
    Medicine
Ascension St. Vincent's
Birmingham, AL, USA

Ina Becker, MD, PhD
Assistant Professor of Psychiatry
Columbia University, Vagelos
    College of Physicians and
    Surgeons
New York, NY, USA

Jay Brenner, MD
Associate Professor
Department of Emergency
    Medicine
SUNY-Upstate Medical University
Syracuse, NY, USA

Jennifer Cullison, PhD
PGY-2 Emergency Medicine
Mercy/St. Vincent Medical Center
Toledo, OH, USA

Lauren J. Curato, DO, FACEP
Assistant Professor
Department of Emergency
    Medicine
Columbia University Vagelos
    College of Physicians and
    Surgeons, New York–
    Presbyterian Hospital
New York, NY, USA

Moira Davenport, MD
Associate Residency Director EM
    Residency
Allegheny General Hospital
Pittsburgh, PA, USA

Arthur R. Derse, MD, JD
Professor and Director
Center for Bioethics and Medical
    Humanities, and Department of
    Emergency Medicine
Medical College of Wisconsin
Milwaukee, WI, USA

Emily Donner, DO
PGY-2 Emergency Medicine
Allegheny General Hospital
Pittsburgh, PA, USA

Clifford Freeman, MD
Clinical Instructor
Department of Emergency
	Medicine
Vanderbilt University
	Medical Center
Nashville, TN, USA

Diane L. Gorgas, MD
Professor and Vice Chair of
	Academic Affairs
Department of Emergency
	Medicine
The Ohio State University
Columbus, OH, USA

Bruce J. Grattan Jr., DO, MS, RD
Resident Physician
Department of Emergency
	Medicine
Bon Secours Mercy/St. Vincent's
	Medical Center
Toledo, OH, USA

Purva Grover, MD, MBA
Medical Director
Department of Emergency
Cleveland Clinic
Cleveland, OH, USA

Max Hensel, MD
Resident Physician
Department of Emergency
Vanderbilt University
	Medical Center
Nashville, TN, USA

David Hoke, MD, MBE
Attending Physician
Department of Emergency
Trident Health System
Summerville, SC, USA

William A. Johnjulio, DO
Chief EM Resident
Allegheny General Hospital
Pittsburgh, PA, USA

Gary Khammahavong, MD
PGY-2 Resident
Department of Emergency
	Medicine
Allegheny General Hospital
Pittsburgh, PA, USA

Mitchell Kosanovich, MD
Assistant Professor
Department of Emergency
	Medicine
Allegheny General Hospital
Pittsburgh, PA, USA

**Chadd K. Kraus, DO,
DrPH, FACEP**
Associate Professor of Emergency
	Medicine, Geisinger
	Commonwealth School of
	Medicine; System Director,
	Emergency Medicine Research;
	Associate Program Director,
	Emergency Medicine Residency
Department of Emergency
	Medicine
Geisinger
Danville, PA, USA

Ryan E. Lawrence, MD
Director, Comprehensive
    Psychiatric Emergency Program
Department of Psychiatry
Columbia University
New York, NY, USA

Nicole McCoin, MD
Keith D. Wrenn Residency
    Program Director and Vice
    Chair for Education
Associate Professor
Department of Emergency
    Medicine
Vanderbilt University
    Medical Center
Nashville, TN, USA

Jillian L. McGrath, MD
Associate Professor
Department of Emergency
    Medicine
The Ohio State University Wexner
    Medical Center
Columbus, OH, USA

Mohamad Moussa, MD, FACEP
Associate Professor
Department of Emergency
    Medicine
University of Toledo College of
    Medicine and Life Sciences
Toledo, OH, USA

Melinda Nguyen, MS, MS-2
University of Toledo College of
    Medicine and Life Sciences
Toledo, OH, USA

Megan A. Panapa, MD
Department of Emergency
    Medicine
Allegheny General Hospital
Pittsburgh, PA, USA

Brent Rau, MD
Attending Physician
Emergency Medicine
Pittsburgh, PA, USA

Alexandra Reinbold, MD
Attending Emergency Physician
Department of Emergency
Providence St. Vincent
Portland, OR, USA

Dana Sacco, MD, MSc
Assistant Professor
Department of Emergency
    Medicine
Columbia University Irving
    Medical Center
New York, NY, USA

Lydia M. Sahlani, MD
Assistant Professor
Department of Emergency
    Medicine
The Ohio State University Wexner
    Medical Center
Columbus, OH, USA

Tyler L. Scaff, MD
Resident Physician
Department of Emergency
    Medicine
Mercy Health St. Vincent
Toledo, OH, USA

Brian L. Springer, MD, FACEP
Associate Professor & Tactical
   Emergency Medicine Director
Department of Emergency
   Medicine
Wright State University
Dayton, OH, USA

Lauren E. Valyo, DO
Department of Emergency
   Medicine
Allegheny General Hospital
Pittsburgh, PA, USA

Carmen Wolfe, MD
Director for Resident Education
Department of Emergency
   Medicine
HCA Healthcare Tristar/Nashville
Nashville, TN, USA

1 Clearly Suicidal and Not Talking

Ina Becker

A 38-year-old married woman is brought to the emergency department by EMS. The EMTs report that she had been talking about having suicidal ideation and wanting to kill herself. She also complains of nausea and vomiting. You have been called to examine her. As you approach her stretcher, you notice that she has long, dark hair that looks matted and somewhat disheveled. She looks pale and is gripping a bowl. As you step to her side, she sits up, bends over the bowl, and throws up liquid material, with a trace of bright red blood. You wait until she is done, and ask her: "Can I help you?" She looks at you for a split second and then puts her finger down her throat and induces vomiting. She then slides down on the stretcher, feet hanging off the edge and begins to moan. She does not answer, and does not look at you. You ask again: "You must feel very nauseous. Is there anything I can do to help you?" She barely looks at you, just groans, and once again puts her finger in her mouth to initiate the gag reflex. She hugs the bowl, throws up clear liquid, and continues to heave. She then turns away from you and stops responding to your offer to help.

What do you do now?

THE PSYCHIATRIC INTERVIEW

The clinical interview is the most important tool in establishing a diagnosis and formulating a treatment plan for any patient with a psychiatric presentation. Despite a multitude of available tests such as blood and urine tests, CT scans, and MRI, it remains usually the most effective tool in the emergency physician's hand, when properly performed. In the majority of cases in the ED, it will lead to the correct diagnosis, or at least will narrow down the differential diagnosis to a few possibilities and thus allow us to begin to formulate a plan and begin treatment. This is important, especially in the ED, where speedy diagnosis and intervention are of the essence.

The ED often tends to be an environment that does not resemble a stereotypical psychiatrist's office at all. Many times, EDs are open spaces, with separations created only by curtains. This provides a setting without any privacy. Most human beings will not want to talk in front of other people about personal details and private concerns. Further, most people will not want to divulge personal information to strangers. In the medical profession, we can at times forget that people look at us as authority figures and trust us with secret and personal information. This is especially true for behavioral health. As emergency physicians, we tend to ask more probing questions than in other specialties, and such questions are often about the most intimate feelings and personal difficulties surrounding identity or success and failure. Patients may feel ashamed about their problems and have internalized thoughts of stigma surrounding "mental problems." Some patients will be concerned with saving face and respectability.

Therefore, when beginning the interview, it is vital to first establish an open atmosphere that communicates respect for the patient. We do this through empathetic, open listening.

Before beginning an interview, several things need to be arranged. The setting has to be safe for the patient and the interviewer and should ideally be private. However, safety takes precedence over privacy. Whenever possible, begin the interview in a setting where other staff or security are present, in case the patient becomes agitated. Once safety has been established, the main part of the interview can proceed.

When approaching a new patient, we may have to first assess if the patient is capable of participating in an interview or needs pharmacologic intervention before the interview can begin. When patients can cooperate with the interview, we begin by introducing ourselves and explaining our role in their evaluation. An open, friendly, but neutral demeanor will go a long way in facilitating a successful interview. Conversational questions may help break the ice. We begin by asking how we can help them. That allows people to speak in their own voice and provide their history how they see it. This is very important. Since our questions are aimed at eliciting patients' understanding of their current situation, we need to give them time to explain how *they see it*. Further, mental/emotional symptoms are more subjective than most physical symptoms. We want to understand the personal, subjective view of the patient's experience.

Our assessment begins before we talk. We assess the person's presentation. Are they well groomed and appropriately dressed? Are they sitting calmly, or is there evidence for psychomotor activity abnormalities? How is their appearance? Do they seem comfortable? Or in pain? Or anxious and panicked? Do they seem to notice their environment, or not? Did someone come with them? All these surrounding details help us, down the line, in making a decision on disposition and treatment.

If patients are unable to provide verbal history or are agitated or highly anxious, information gathering may initially mean drawing blood tests and doing a physical exam, listening to the content of their spontaneous, disorganized utterances, or yelling and cursing, which allows for at least some insight into their internal physical and emotional states and thought processes. For example, someone in the midst of a panic attack may benefit from an injection of a short-acting benzodiazepine.

The initial goal of a psychiatric interview in the ED is to arrive at a decision whether to discharge, admit, or hold for further observation in the ED, and to stabilize the acute crisis. It is important to resist the natural human tendency to quickly make a decision moments after we meet someone; instead, we should gather as much information as necessary to make a *good* decision. The second objective of the initial interview is to arrive at a diagnosis, which will then suggest a treatment plan.

The initial assessment may not even include a dialog, as in the example above. What we have learned so far from the woman is that she is in no condition to leave, as she is likely nauseated, definitely vomiting, and not able to talk in a coherent manner. She may feel suicidal and have made an attempt to kill herself by overdosing. For her, we will proceed with a medical workup, physical exam, blood work that includes toxicology screens, and an EKG to search for medical causes of her current state. We will definitely keep her in the ED for further observation. In patients who cannot be properly interviewed, it is often beneficial to stop by their bedside every hour or so to observe their condition and behavior.

If the patient appears anxious and answers with only a few words without elaborating, we may want to provide more structure and begin asking simple questions about geographic and general information, such as address, relationships, and medical history. Anxious and psychotic patients are often not able to provide information in a coherent manner and may appreciate being able to answer simple questions. For patients who are psychotic or manic, listening to their spontaneous talk will often give us valuable information about their thought processes. As mentioned above, during the initial stage of the interview, we want to establish an empathetic rapport with the patient and ask open-ended questions, to allow her to trust us with her care.

IMPORTANT ELEMENTS OF THE PSYCHIATRIC HISTORY AND REVIEW OF SYSTEMS

After eliciting the presenting chief complaint, we will ideally have to gather a complete history, as outlined in Box 1.1. A complete psychiatric interview will include answers to most of the elements of the Review of Systems, listed in Table 1.1. It must include a review of the patient's mood and anxiety, and thought process and content (disordered thought forms are numerous and are signs of psychoses and delirium), perceptual disturbances, and cognition. Ideally, it will cautiously touch on a patient's trauma history, without inquiring about any details that may be triggering flashbacks or dissociation. The discussion of a past history of trauma or abuse is one of the most delicate parts of the initial interview. These experiences are deeply painful and intimate. It is generally best to explain to patients that they will not have to discuss any details of past traumas, but that it will help us help them if we know that they have had significant traumatic experiences. People generally have no difficulty speaking of car accidents or war trauma,

BOX 1.1 **Questionnaire for Psychiatric Interview**

Identifying information
    Brought in by
    Contact for collateral history
Chief complaint
History of present illness
    Stressors leading to visit, why now?
    Support system
    Children, ages, whereabouts
Substance use
    Current/past, which drugs
    History of alcohol withdrawal?
Past psychiatric history and diagnoses
    Hospitalizations
    Outpatient treatment history
    Medication trials
    Suicide attempts
    Non-suicidal self-injurious behaviors
Past medical history
    Allergies
    Current medications
    Current supplements/vitamins
Social history
    Born where
    Highest education/work experience
    Housing/homeless
    Employment
    Partner/married?
Mental status exam
    Grooming
    Attitude
    Eye contact
    Psychomotor activity
    Speech quality
    Mood/affect
    Thought form
    Hallucinations
    Delusions
    Suicidal
    Homicidal
    Insight
    Judgment

BOX 1.1 Continued

Cognitive exam
    Level of alertness
    Orientation
    Attention
    Immediate recall
    Short-term memory
    Long-term memory
    Abstractions
    Naming
    Insight/judgment
Share alerts
    Homeless
    Access to guns
    Violence
    Suicide attempt/non-suicidal self-injurious behavior
    Chronic non-adherence
    Fall risk
    Frequent ED visits
    Withdrawal/complications
Medical comorbidities
Vital signs
Bloods: CBC, BMP, LFT, TSH
Urine: UA, urine toxicology, beta-hCG
Head imaging
Diagnostic impression
Plan
History of violence, legal history, guns?

whereas survivors of physical and sexual abuse, often perpetrated by family members, will often feel ashamed and guilt-ridden.

With a cooperative patient, the exam will include a history of past psychiatric illness, treatment, history of past hospitalizations, ED visits, suicide attempts, history of violence or arrests, and adherence to medications. If medications were tried, how they worked and who prescribed them should be noted. Legal history, including history of arrests, and access to firearms are important to inquire about.

Suicidal ideation is one of the foremost reasons for people to seek help in the ED, and we are tasked with assessing the seriousness of their ideation.

TABLE 1.1 **Psychiatric Review of Systems**

Mania	Distractibility, irresponsibility, grandiosity, flight of ideas, activity increase, sleep deficit, talkativeness
Depression	Sleep, interest, guilt, energy, concentration, appetite, psychomotor, suicidal ideation, worthlessness, helplessness
Psychosis	Auditory/visual/tactile/somatic hallucinations, delusions (paranoid, grandiose, religious, somatic), thought insertion or withdrawal, thought disorders (illogical, looseness of association, flight of ideas), ideas of reference
Suicide/self-injurious behavior	Ideation, passive/active, intent, which plans, protective factors, what stops you, past attempts, non-suicidal self-injurious behavior (cutting, burning, sexual acting out/promiscuity, recklessness, substance use)
Homicide/violence	Ideation, intent, plan, nonspecific/particular person, past fights or violence
Anxiety	Generalized/episodic, physical/mental, obsessive thoughts, compulsive rituals
Trauma	History of abuse/traumatic events, avoid detailed discussion, history of dissociation
Orientation/cognitive exam/judgment	Level of alertness, attention, memory (immediate, short-term, long-term), visuospatial abilities, naming, language comprehension, abstractions, executive functioning, estimate of intelligence (normal range/not)

We must directly and openly explore the details of suicidal ideation, intent, and plan and past suicidal behavior/attempts.

Lastly, most people who seek psychiatric help in the ED are in genuine and severe distress and want help. They will be as truthful as they can and explain their problem as best they can. But there are a few people who come to the ED with a particular agenda, seeking secondary gain, and presenting with malingering symptoms. Examples of these are the homeless person who wants to sleep in the ED for a night, get food, and take a shower, or others who complain of unverifiable pain, seeking opiate prescriptions. It is often difficult to detect malingering in a first interview. Nonverbal aspects of communication can be helpful in detecting manufactured versus real symptoms. For example, someone who is psychotic will appear internally preoccupied and distressed by what derogatory voices are telling him/her. In contrast, a person who is malingering, who claims to hear voices without actually hearing them, will likely appear to be relatively at ease, although the words used to describe their situations may be the same. Someone who is hungry will be more focused on getting food than in describing the details of his/her chief complaint of suicidal ideation. Even if the presenting complaint is not the actual reason for the ED visit, everybody deserves to be respected and heard. Social workers may be able to help in cases of malingering for food and shelter, where medical intervention cannot.

Many times, it is difficult to complete the entire review of systems in the ED setting, where patients are often highly distressed. As a general rule, people will bring up issues that are most important to them and that distress them the most. Details of a complete psychiatric interview can wait until the initial crisis has been stabilized. For example, it will likely be futile to try and ask paranoid patients about obsessive rituals and traumatic experiences, as they will interpret these questions through a psychotic, paranoid lens and find them to be more reasons for paranoia.

CASE RESOLUTION

For the woman in our case example, the result of the blood tests provided a first clue for understanding her crisis. Her glucose level was 545, BP 124/78, pulse 110. Toxicology screens were negative. She was given insulin and fluids. She was also given a total of 4 mg lorazepam IV to stop her from self-inducing vomiting. Her mother arrived soon after this was initiated and provided more history.

Her mother informed us that the patient had been extremely anxious at the prospect of beginning a new job at a local supermarket on the day of presentation to the ED. She had a history of extreme bouts of anxiety and panic attacks ever since her husband left her a year ago. The patient was in treatment with a local psychiatrist and was being prescribed venlafaxine 225 mg and hydroxyzine 25 mg, as needed for anxiety attacks.

She had discontinued her home insulin and antidepressant on the day prior to presentation and had started eating whatever she wanted, including binging on sweets. Her diagnoses were type 1 diabetes; anxiety; depression; eating disorder, bulimic type; and borderline personality disorder traits. In the past, she had been admitted to a medical floor of another hospital, where she needed to be restrained to prevent her from inducing vomiting while receiving IV fluids.

Her glucose level normalized with treatment, and she was restarted on venlafaxine 75 mg, which relieved any withdrawal symptoms related to her serotonin–norepinephrine reuptake inhibitor (SNRI). She continued to receive regular doses of lorazepam. After several days on a medical unit, she stopped feeling anxious, stopped vomiting, and provided a history. After finding out that her new boyfriend had been cheating on her, she felt like she did not care about anything and wanted to die, so she stopped her medications. She still felt she no longer wanted to be alive. After medical stabilization was completed, she was transferred to the inpatient psychiatry unit for further treatment.

KEY POINTS TO REMEMBER

- A person who is not talking is not safe for discharge.
- The severity of suicidality and homicidality needs to be assessed before discharge can be considered.
- A good evaluation may occur in several parts and will improve the treatment plan.

Further Reading

American Psychiatric Association. *Practice Guidelines for the Psychiatric Evaluations of Adults.* 3rd ed. Arlington, VA: American Psychiatric Association; 2016.
Hart M, Lewine RRJ. Rethinking thought disorder. *Schizophren Bull.* 2017;43(3):514–522.

Kyser JG, Diner BC, Raulston GW. A practical approach to the assessment and management of psychiatric emergencies. *Jefferson J Psychiatry*. 1989;7(2): Article 13.

Meyers J, Stein S. The psychiatric interview in the emergency department. *Emerg Clin North Am*. 2000;18(2):173–183.

Nordgaard J, Sass LA, Parnas J. The psychiatric interview: Validity, structure, and subjectivity. *Eur Arch Psychiatry Clin Neurosci*. 2013;263(4):353–364.

Sullivan HS. *The Psychiatric Interview*. New York: Norton; 1970.

2 We Need Labs and an EKG

Chadd K. Kraus

A 47-year-old female presents to the ED for worsening anxiety and a plan for suicide by jumping off a bridge. The patient is known to the ED staff from prior visits for anxiety, depression, and suicidal thoughts. She is in her normal state of health, with no other symptoms. Vital signs are HR 98, BP 158/86, RR 18, temp 97.9°F, and SpO_2 98% on room air. The emergency physician performs a history and physical exam. She determines that the patient requires inpatient psychiatric evaluation and treatment. The emergency physician calls the on-call psychiatrist at the nearest psychiatric facility with available inpatient beds to admit the patient. The on-call psychiatrist requests that the emergency physician order an EKG, cardiac enzymes, a complete metabolic panel, and a CBC, as well as treating the patient's elevated BP. The emergency physician reports to the psychiatrist that the medical screening exam is complete and the patient is medically appropriate for psychiatric evaluation.

What do you do now?

PSYCHIATRIC SCREENING EXAM

Frequently, psychiatric facilities have policies that require certain information (e.g., lab test results) or request specific medical evaluations before accepting patients from EDs. The emergency physician must decide how to address these requests, including whether they are necessary to accomplish the needs of the patient. In meeting the Emergency Medical Treatment and Active Labor Act (EMTALA) obligation to provide a medical screening exam, the minimal elements necessary in the medical evaluation of patients with psychiatric complaints in the ED are a thorough history and physical examination, including vital signs and mental status exam.[1] Patients presenting to the ED with psychiatric chief complaints can be adequately screened and cleared for admission to inpatient psychiatry with history and physical alone.[2,3]

It is unlikely that laboratory tests or other diagnostic results will change the clinical course or disposition for the patient from psychiatric admission to medical admission. One study suggested that among "patients presenting to the ED with a psychiatric chief complaint and no physical complaints, abnormal vital signs, or abnormal physical exam findings [there is] less than 1 percent probability that an abnormal laboratory study will change their disposition from a psychiatric admission to a medical admission."[4] Further, routine, urine-based drug screens in this patient population are not recommended.[5]

The American College of Emergency Physicians (ACEP) recommends against routine laboratory testing for the evaluation of patients presenting to the ED with psychiatric symptoms. In its clinical policy on the care of patients with psychiatric symptoms, ACEP states, "In the alert adult patient presenting to the emergency department with acute psychiatric symptoms . . . Do not routinely order laboratory testing on patients with acute psychiatric symptoms. Use medical history, previous psychiatric diagnoses, and physician examination to guide testing."[5] Routine laboratory tests in patients with "benign histories and normal physical exams have a low likelihood of clinical significant laboratory findings."[6]

There are potential negative, unintended consequences of routine laboratory testing in the evaluation of patients with psychiatric symptoms presenting to the ED. Increases in ED length of stay have been reported with such routine laboratory testing.[7] This increased length of stay is potentially a detrimental consequence for the patient who requires timely psychiatric care. There is also the potential for increased morbidity and mortality in the misdiagnosis of medical illnesses in patients with acute psychiatric needs.[8] Therefore, not only are routine, screening laboratory tests largely unnecessary in patients with psychiatric symptoms presenting to the ED, but these tests might also have negative consequences for the patient.

Laboratory testing is not always contraindicated in this population of patients. Certain features, particularly in agitated patients, including abnormal vital signs, abnormal physical examination results, signs and symptoms of alcohol or drug intoxication or withdrawal, and decreased attention or alertness, are suggestive of medical etiologies of symptoms and require further diagnostic investigation.[9] In limited circumstances, an ED might fulfill a request by a psychiatric facility without phlebotomy services to perform a lab draw, although such requests should not delay patient transfer to the definitive care provided at a psychiatric facility, and results can be communicated later to the receiving facility.[1,10]

There has been a move away from the traditionally used phrase "medical clearance" for the ED evaluation of psychiatric patients. Instead, following appropriate and adequate medical evaluation in the ED, a "transfer note should accompany the patient indicating the patient is medically stable and appropriate for treatment in a psychiatric setting."[1]

Ideally a "brief cognitive exam should include assessment of attention, executive function, orientation, and recent memory."[1] Specific screening tools have been developed to identify patients at higher risk for medical conditions,[11] although these are not widely used, and more concise examinations can be used by emergency physicians to determine whether a patient is medically appropriate for psychiatric evaluation.

CASE RESOLUTION

The patient in this case is asymptomatic and has no clinical evidence to suggest acute end-organ damage related to hypertension. While emergent evaluation for end-organ damage is warranted, medical treatment of asymptomatic hypertension in the ED is usually not recommended.[12] The emergency physician should determine if the patient's hypertension is newly discovered or a chronic issue. If an adequate history and physical exam suggests no acute end-organ damage, the emergency physician should discuss with the patient the importance of BP control on an outpatient basis.

In this case, the emergency physician should communicate clearly with the accepting psychiatrist regarding the asymptomatic hypertension and reinforce that based on history (including the patient's past psychiatric-related ED visits) and exam, the patient would not require routine laboratory or other diagnostic (e.g., EKG) testing for admission for psychiatric evaluation. The emergency physician should also be cognizant that many psychiatric facilities have limited capabilities for managing medical issues. If the psychiatrist requests laboratory testing because the facility does not have services to obtain labs, that request could be fulfilled, but not at the expense of delayed transfer while awaiting results. The patient's acute psychiatric needs should be prioritized and chronic medical conditions such as hypertension can be addressed in an outpatient setting, without detriment to timely management, including care in a specialized setting, of an acute psychiatric need.

KEY POINTS TO REMEMBER

- Patients presenting to the ED with psychiatric complaints should have an evaluation for alternate etiologies of their symptoms if indicated.
- A history of psychiatric illness, normal vital signs, normal alertness and orientation, and absence of medical complaints make a medical etiology for symptoms highly unlikely.
- Transfer to definitive psychiatric care should not be delayed to obtain medical diagnostic tests in an otherwise clinically stable patient presenting to the ED with a psychiatric chief complaint.

References

1. Wilson MP, Nordstrom K, Anderson EL, et al. American Association for Emergency Psychiatry Task Force on Medical Clearance of Adult Psychiatric Patients. Part II: Controversies over medical assessment, and consensus recommendations. *West J Emerg Med*. 2017;18(4):640–646.

2. Janiak BD, Atteberry S. Medical clearance of the psychiatric patient in the emergency department. *J Emerg Med*. 2012;43(5):866–870.

3. Korn CS, Currier GW, Henderson SO. "Medical clearance" of psychiatric patients without medical complaints in the emergency department. *J Emerg Med*. 2000;18(2):173–176.

4. Kagel KE, Smith M, Latyshenko IV, et al. Effects of mandatory screening labs in directing the disposition of the apparently healthy psychiatric patient in the emergency department. *US Army Med Dep J*. 2017;(2–17):18–24.

5. American College of Emergency Physicians (ACEP). Clinical policy: Critical issues in the diagnosis and management of the adult psychiatric patient in the emergency department. 2017. https://www.acep.org/contentassets/04e7623d4991 457bbcd9a53a40ba427d/cp-adultpsychiatricpatient-1.pdf

6. Amin M, Wang J. Routine laboratory testing to evaluate for medical illness in psychiatric patients in the emergency department is largely unrevealing. *West J Emerg Med*. 2009;10(2):97–100.

7. Donofrio JJ, Santillanes G, McCammack BD, et al. Clinical utility of screening laboratory tests in pediatric psychiatric patients presenting to the emergency department for medical clearance. *Ann Emerg Med*. 2014;63(6):666–675.

8. Tucci V, Siever K, Matorin A, Moukaddam N. Down the rabbit hole: Emergency department medical clearance of patients with psychiatric or behavioral emergencies. *Emerg Med Clin North Am*. 2015;33(4):721–737.

9. Nordstrom K, Zun LS, Wilson MP, et al. Medical evaluation and triage of the agitated patient: Consensus statement of the American Association for Emergency Psychiatry Project BETA Medical Evaluation Workgroup. *West J Emerg Med*. 2012;13(1):3–10.

10. Thrasher TW, Rolli M, Redwood RS, et al. "Medical clearance" of patients with acute mental health needs in the emergency department: A literature review and practice recommendations. *WMJ*. 2019;118(4):156–163.

11. Shah SJ, Fiorito M, McNamara RM. A screening tool to medically clear psychiatric patients in the emergency department. *J Emerg Med*. 2012;43(5):871–875.

12. American College of Emergency Physicians (ACEP). Clinical policy: Critical issues in the evaluation and management of adult patients in the emergency department with asymptomatic elevated blood pressure. 2013. https://www.acep.org/globalassets/new-pdfs/clinical-policies/asympt-hypert2-final-bod-approved-2013.pdf

3 Naked and Afraid

Tyler L. Scaff

A 46-year-old woman with past medical history of homelessness and paranoid-type schizophrenia presents to the ED via EMS after being found wandering in the street and yelling at passing cars. She is a new patient to this hospital and no further history is available. On arrival, she is visibly agitated and states that the FBI is coming to kill her, and that they have been monitoring her movements for "years." She states that they put a "computer chip" in her brain to track her movements and listen to her thoughts, and she hears them telling her to hurt people and herself. She is unable to answer questions about medication, past medical history, surgeries, allergies, or social history. When EMS attempts to leave, she becomes more agitated and states that the paramedics are her "protection." Despite attempts by ED staff to calm her down she punches the attending physician and attempts to flee the hospital.

What do you do now?

AGITATION IN THE ED

This case, taken from an actual case I witnessed during my sub-internship in Oklahoma, demonstrates that agitated patients may at times be unable to be reasoned with. But this is not always the case. In this chapter, we will explore the many different causes of agitation in the ED, how to mitigate these factors, and how to manage the patient whose agitation has snowballed into threats and violence.

Something we often forget as ED practitioners is that the ED is an extremely uncomfortable, unnatural environment for patients. Picture it for yourself: You are resting at home late at night when suddenly a pain wakes you from sleep. You come to the ED for evaluation, and several people take vital signs from you and ask you a litany of questions. Then you are rushed into a room with a thin curtain drawn to separate you from the rest of the department. Outside, the lights are always on. The department is often abuzz with a chorus of beeping monitors, rumbling floor cleaners, energetic staff, overhead pages, crying children, and patients moaning or downright screaming in pain. There is a strong, foul odor emanating from the room next to you. You are feeling quite cold and naked in your ugly hospital gown. Staff will be in every couple of hours or more to take your vital signs, puncture your skin with needles, ask you more questions, and take you to various locations for further workup. All the while, you remain in pain. It is not surprising that some people who may ordinarily be amicable grow restless and occasionally violent in such a stressful atmosphere.

In the case described at the beginning of this chapter, it was clear that this person with a known history of paranoid schizophrenia was already in the middle of an acute psychotic episode. She was quickly brought in to the bright and noisy ED during a hot Oklahoma afternoon, surrounded by staff members who were understandably concerned with her behavior and asking many questions. This sudden increase in stimulation further escalated her behavior and she began shouting that she wanted to leave. During this time, the only two people she even slightly knew (the paramedics) stepped out of the room after giving report. Though this patient may have been better controlled in another, less demanding environment, the pressure and unfamiliarity of the ED sent her reeling into a panic.

However, this patient was not the only person who came unprepared; so were the staff. Often this ED received patients with little advance notice; the only two staff members near the patient at the time of her arrival were the resident and attending physician—no nurses, no security. With quicker access to restraints and sedative medications, it is likely that this patient could have been controlled before she posed a danger to herself and others.

MASLOW'S HIERARCHY OF NEEDS

Though this case explores a situation in which a patient cannot be reasoned with, much of the success in controlling agitated patients lies in preventing them becoming agitated in the first place. For this reason, we explore prevention and de-escalation strategies following Maslow's hierarchy of needs, a well-known psychological construct that describes a structure of five categories of need. One builds upon the other; without the former, the latter cannot be achieved. These categories, from basic to advanced, are as follows:

1. **Physiological needs.** This includes food, water, shelter, air, sleep, clothing, and ability to use their senses normally (i.e., having glasses or hearing aids within reach). During every patient encounter, ask yourself: What could you do to make them feel more comfortable? For example, how long have they been NPO? What is the environment of their exam room like? Do they have clean clothes? A blanket? And even though you may be awake during your night shift, would it be reasonable to allow your patient to sleep in the wee hours of the morning?

2. **Safety needs.** This includes personal security, resources, physical well-being, and personal property. Does the patient have access to his/her phone, keys, wallet, etc., or at least know the location of them? Are they in pain, and if so, would they benefit from pain medication? And for those who may be in acute psychosis, feeling threatened by their hallucinations or delusions, would they benefit from an antipsychotic?

3. **Love and belonging.** This includes family, friends, and the sense of connection one feels with others. The easiest and most effective

way for an emergency provider to impart this is to sit down in the room. Take time to understand the patient's concerns, and in this same vein, watch what you and staff members say outside the room. Patients have often heard conversations between staff members using such trigger phrases as "drug-seeking," "malingering," or "crazy." It doesn't matter if they are talking about that patient; often just hearing these words can cause a deep rift between the patient and the caregiver.

4. **Esteem.** This includes respect, self-esteem, and the freedom to make one's own decisions. In the ED, that may refer to asking questions as important as whether or not they wish to be admitted, or as trivial as what kind of juice they would like. Depending on the individual's circumstance and decision-making ability, there is often room for patient preference. Conflicts can sometimes be avoided entirely by providing the patient with autonomy that he/she has the decision-making capacity to handle.

5. **Self-actualization.** One's aspiration to be the most that one can be.

Understanding this structure can benefit an emergency provider's ability to handle agitated patients tremendously. Too often the well-meaning provider may attempt to have a discussion about the agitated patient's concerns when in fact the patient is focused on more basic needs, such as hunger, fatigue, breathing problems, or pain. Considering these needs first may serve as de-escalation in and of itself.

Now suppose that you have tried all of the above, and your patient is unable to be calmed. We often reach then for sedatives and restraints, which is not unreasonable, but it is important to understand that patients can also be participants in their own de-escalation. I have been surprised by the patients who actually *want* to calm down and are willing to take PO or IV medications to relax them. For these people, oral lorazepam (1–2 mg), diphenhydramine (50 mg), or IV haloperidol (2 mg) is a reasonable option. Bear in mind that patients with long QT syndrome are at risk of ventricular arrhythmias with high doses of antipsychotic medications (see "Further Reading"). A prior EKG is helpful. Though IM ziprasidone carries a higher QTc prolongation than haloperidol, it is less likely to cause the dreaded tardive dyskinesia (see "Further Reading"). Ultimately, in the completely unreasonable patient, the priority is the safety of all involved. Security should be called to the bedside long before restraints are required, and sedative medications should be ready to administer. High-risk patients should be searched for weapons and placed on continuous surveillance until the threat is neutralized. Do not forget that, after administration of sedating medications, the patient must be watched for respiratory or cardiovascular depression.

CASE RESOLUTION

Unfortunately, things did not go as planned in this situation. The patient, in her desperation to catch up to the paramedics, punched an attending physician who attempted to stop her. The attending yelled for security personnel, who were delayed in response because they were wrapped up with another combative patient. The second-year ED resident—and I am not making this up—wrapped the flailing patient in a bear hug from behind and took her to the ground. Still screaming, the patient kicked out with all four limbs and reached behind her head, attempting to claw at the resident. Security arrived and relieved the resident, placing the patient in a five-point hold prone on the ground while a nurse administered an IM medication combination consisting of 10 mg haloperidol, 2 mg lorazepam, and 100 mg diphenhydramine. It still took several minutes for the adrenaline-charged patient to calm down enough to be properly restrained supine in a bed. The patient was immobilized in a cervical collar and a comprehensive trauma survey was performed, including non-contrast CT head, CT cervical spine, and bedside extended focused assessment with sonography for trauma (E-FAST) examination. The survey, urine drug screen, and ED toxicology panel were all negative. After several hours of monitoring, the patient woke up enough to be safely discharged to a psychiatric facility.

> **KEY POINTS TO REMEMBER**
>
> · Know their needs: Maslow's hierarchy of needs starts with physiological (food, hydration, ability to see/hear normally), followed by safety (access to personal items, pain medication),

belonging (family members, physician–patient relationship), esteem (clarifying the patient's wishes), and self-actualization.
. An ounce of prevention: Consider the basic needs of your patient using Maslow's hierarchy as your guide. A hungry, tired, overstimulated, isolated patient is a recipe for aggression.
. A pound of cure: When aggression is unavoidable, prioritize security, sedation, and supervision.

Further Reading

American College of Emergency Physicians. *Tintinalli's Emergency Medicine Manual*. 9th ed. New York: McGraw-Hill Medical; 2020:1933–1966.

Ananth J, Burgoyne KS, Niz D, Smith M. Tardive dyskinesia in two patients treated with ziprasidone. *J Psychiatry Neurosci*. 2004;29(6):467–469.

Cherry K. The five levels of Maslow's hierarchy of needs. VeryWellMind. 2015. http://psychology.about.com/od/theoriesofpersonality/a/hierarchyneeds.htm

Washington NB, Brahm MC, Kissack J. Which psychotropics carry the greatest risk of QTc prolongation? *Current Psychiatry*. 2012;11(10):36–39.

4 Take a Chill Pill

Lydia M. Sahlani and Jillian L. McGrath

A 26-year-old male is brought to the ED by the police for aggressive behavior. Police report that they were called by the patient's family reporting that he threatened them with a knife. He has a history of depression and substance abuse. The family noted several weeks of increasingly paranoid and bizarre behavior. The police report that the patient became violent and resisted officers when they arrived on scene, necessitating the use of physical restraint prior to arrival. The patient appears disheveled and is thrashing around on the gurney while your security staff apply physical restraints. He is alert, diaphoretic, and verbally threatening security and nursing staff. He has superficial cuts on both hands, but no other obvious signs of trauma. You are unable to obtain vital signs due to the patient's level of agitation. You attempt to verbally de-escalate the situation in order to gather patient history, yet he refuses to answer any questions and continues to yell profanities and threats of harm to you and your staff.

What do you do now?

CHEMICAL RESTRAINT IN THE AGITATED PATIENT

Acutely agitated patients pose significant risk of harm to themselves or others if not rapidly assessed and managed. Such patients are frequently brought to the ED with chief complaints of "altered mental status" or "psychiatric illness." The etiology of acute agitation is varied; organic medical conditions, drug effects, and decompensated psychiatric conditions can all present in this way. In order for ED physicians and other providers to appropriately care for these patients, a systematic approach is needed. This patient in the case poses a significant challenge in management. His behavior precludes front-line personnel, including law enforcement and medical providers, from promptly assessing his medical and psychological state. If his agitation is not managed promptly, it will prevent his medical team from offering timely evaluation of the underlying causes and tailoring medical therapy to his needs.

This case highlights techniques that are commonly employed to manage acutely agitated patients, including verbal de-escalation and physical or chemical restraint. When it is appropriate to the circumstance, verbal de-escalation should be attempted first. Using non-threatening body language and clear and calm speech may help diffuse some situations. This method failed in this case. Thus, alternative options such as physical or chemical restraint must be considered. It is crucial for the physician or provider to assess the patient immediately when escalating to other methods of management. In this case, the patient poses a serious threat to others and adequate assessment and treatment cannot be accomplished in his current state. The provider should identify that the use of chemical restraint is necessary. It should be noted that providers should always document the rationale for use of physical and chemical restraint, given the significant infringement on the patient's autonomy. Security staff and police are often used to physically restrain the patient while measures are taken to administer chemical restraint. Manual restraint is best achieved using one person to secure each limb and one person to monitor the patient's head and airway while medications for chemical restraint are prepared. Thorough assessment, including patient vital signs and EKG, although typically assessed prior to sedation, are deferred until they can safely be obtained after acutely agitated patients are sedated. The need for physical restraint should consistently be reassessed and then eliminated as soon as it is safe to do so.

When ordering chemical sedation, first consider the appropriate route of administration. PO medications can be trialed if the patient is cooperative enough and the longer time to onset is deemed safe. IV options are favorable given predictable absorption and onset times, although it is rarely feasible to obtain IV access in a scenario like this case. As a result, IM medications are often preferred initially. Patient characteristics, such as level of agitation, age, weight, medical history, and medications (including drug dependence or response to prior sedating medications), should be considered when determining the best medication and dosage for chemical sedation. Effective pharmacologic options that are easily accessible in most emergency settings are benzodiazepines, antipsychotics, and ketamine.

Combining benzodiazepines and typical antipsychotics (most frequently lorazepam and haloperidol) is common and considered the first-line choice for chemical restraint in the undifferentiated ED patient due to widespread availability, synergistic effect, and safety profile. Readily available benzodiazepines include lorazepam, midazolam, and diazepam. Lorazepam is the most commonly used due to its rapid onset and overall low drug interaction risk as compared to other benzodiazepines (it is less affected by drug interactions or liver disease because it does not involve CYP450 metabolism). Typical dosing for lorazepam is 1 to 2 mg PO, SL, IM, or IV every 2 to 6 hours, although individual patient response to benzodiazepines varies. Midazolam has rapid onset but is shorter acting than lorazepam and may require repeat dosing. Midazolam has been shown to achieve more effective sedation at 15 minutes than haloperidol, ziprasidone, and perhaps olanzapine. It is typically dosed IM 5 to 10 mg or IV 2.5 to 5 mg every 3 minutes. Diazepam has slower IV onset and IM dosing is not recommended due to poor absorption; it is dosed 5 mg every 3 minutes, up to 30 mg. It should be noted that the use of benzodiazepines alone is implicated in greater need for repeat dosing, as well as the increased likelihood of primarily respiratory adverse events. Benzodiazepines should be used with caution in the elderly and patients with underlying respiratory disease or compromise.

Antipsychotics, both typical and atypical, can be used for chemical restraint. In addition, they may help control psychotic symptoms. Common typical antipsychotics include droperidol and haloperidol. These medications carry a risk of QT prolongation. QT intervals greater than 500 msec can lead to ventricular arrhythmias, particularly torsades de pointes.

Although considered controversial, owing to a black box warning, repeat dosing should be carried out with some caution. Ideally, obtain serial EKG or cardiac monitoring to evaluate this potential effect. Both droperidol and haloperidol can be administered IM or IV. Droperidol is dosed 5 to 10 mg IM or 2.5 to 5 mg IV, up to 20 mg. Haloperidol is dosed 2.5 to 5 mg IV every 2 to 3 minutes, up to 10 mg. It is commonly dosed at 5 mg IM, and repeated every hour until sedation is achieved, up to 20 mg/day. Some atypical antipsychotics such as olanzapine have been studied extensively with regard to chemical restraint. Olanzapine has been shown to have a superior sedation effect in agitated ED patients when compared with haloperidol; however, it has a longer duration of action and is synergistic with other CNS depressants. It is dosed 10 mg IM or 5 mg IV every 5 minutes, with a maximum of 20 mg IV. Some studies show that PO risperidone is as effective as IM haloperidol or the combination therapy of haloperidol and lorazepam. Other atypical antipsychotics such as ziprasidone and aripiprazole have not been extensively studied in emergency medicine literature but have a role in differentiated patients with schizophrenia or mania.

Ketamine is a good option for patients who have failed attempts at chemical restraint or for initial sedation in severely agitated patients. Notably, this medication does not cause respiratory depression. It rarely causes laryngospasm and may require airway management. Thus, it should be used with caution in patients with hypertension and tachycardia, as well as those with schizophrenia (as it can exacerbate symptoms). Due to its relatively good side-effect profile and rapid onset, this medication is often used in prehospital settings. It is dosed 1 mg/kg IV or 5 mg/kg IM.

Table 4.1 highlights commonly used IM medications for chemical restraint.

CASE RESOLUTION

In this case, it is important to quickly identify that this patient poses a threat to his own safety and that of his care providers. The provider should document attempts at verbal de-escalation and the need for physical restraint. Ultimately, rapid chemical restraint is necessary to ensure safety. In this scenario, the history provided regarding paranoia and bizarre behavior raises concern for psychiatric disturbance or substance abuse. Considering

TABLE 4.1 **Common IM medications used for chemical restraint**

Drug	Dose (IM)	Onset (min)	Potential effects
Benzodiazepines			
Lorazepam	2 mg	15–30	Sedation, respiratory depression
Midazolam	5 mg	10–15	
Typical Antipsychotics			
Haloperidol	5–10 mg	10–20	Extrapyramidal symptoms, prolonged QTc
Droperidol	5–10 mg	10–30	Extrapyramidal symptoms, cardiac dysrhythmia
Atypical Antipsychotic			
Olanzapine	10 mg	15–30	Sedation, respiratory depression
Other			
Ketamine	5 mg/kg	3–5	Laryngospasm, hypertension, delirium or hallucination

the patient's age, medical history, and current presentation, the use of a benzodiazepine in conjunction with a typical antipsychotic will likely result in safe, rapid chemical restraint. The patient would benefit from an EKG to assess QT interval, as well as vital signs and laboratory workup to identify any medical causes of agitation as soon as it is safe to obtain this information. Monitoring and reassessment while in the ED should be frequent in order to minimize physical restraint and evaluate for any adverse effects of chemical restraint.

KEY POINTS TO REMEMBER

· Agitated patients frequently present to the ED.
· Verbal de-escalation techniques are preferred in initial management of agitated patients whenever safe, but they may prove to be unsuccessful.

- Physical and chemical restraint techniques are often required for safety when treating acutely agitated patients in the ED.
- Common medications used to achieve chemical restraint include benzodiazepines, antipsychotics, and ketamine.
- Factors to consider when ordering chemical restraint include patient factors such as age, weight, and medical conditions as well as the likely underlying cause of agitation.
- Monitoring and reassessment is crucial to ensure patient safety and appropriately treat underlying conditions.

Further Reading

Battaglia J, Moss S, Rush J, et al. Haloperidol, lorazepam, or both for psychotic agitation: A multicenter, prospective, double-blind, emergency department study. *Am J Emerg Med*. 1997;15:335–340.

Godwin SA, Burton JH, Gerardo CJ, et al. Clinical policy: Procedural sedation and analgesia in the emergency department. *Ann Emerg Med*. 2014;63(2):247–258.

Hopper AB, Vilke GM, Castillo EM, et al. Ketamine use for acute agitation in the emergency department. *J Emerg Med*. 2015;48(6):712–719.

Isbister GK, Calver LA, Page CB, et al. Randomized controlled trial of intramuscular droperidol versus midazolam for violence and acute behavioral disturbance: The DORM study. *Ann Emerg Med*. 2010;56(4):392–401.

Klein LR, Driver BE, Miner JR, et al. Intramuscular midazolam, olanzapine, ziprasidone, or haloperidol for treating acute agitation in the emergency department. *Ann Emerg Med*. 2018;72(4):374–385.

Kroczak S, Kirby A, Gunja N. Chemical agents for the sedation of agitated patients in the ED: A systematic review. *Am J Emerg Med*. 2016;34(12):2426–2431.

Rund DA, Ewing JD, Mitzel K, Votolato N. The use of intramuscular benzodiazepines and antipsychotic agents in the treatment of acute agitation or violence in the emergency department. *J Emerg Med*. 2006;31(3):317–324.

5 Compassionate Restraint in the ED

Clifford Freeman and Carmen Wolfe

EMS brings a 28-year-old male to your ED after he was found walking down the middle of a local road yelling at cars. Paramedics report that the patient is well known to them and has a documented history of schizophrenia with frequent bouts of psychosis. They note a history of combative behavior, but so far today he has been cooperative, allowing them to obtain vital signs and perform a limited initial assessment, which revealed no evidence of trauma. His vital signs were recorded with BP 147/68, HR 112, RR 18, SpO_2 98% on room air. A blood glucose was obtained and was 87. After being taken to his assessment room, the patient becomes verbally abusive with his nurse, who calls for security to the room given her concern for his escalating behavior. As you arrive to the doorway, the patient is screaming, "Let me go or I will kill all of you!" You ask him what you can do to improve his situation and offer him some food and a drink, but he continues to yell. He then grabs the nurse by the arm and attempts to punch her.

What do you do now?

PHYSICAL RESTRAINTS IN THE ED

Options for Managing Violence in the ED

The initial approach in the management of a violent or agitated patient should include attempts at verbal de-escalation. If possible, create a calm and quiet environment for the patient encounter, while still giving proper attention to staff safety and ensuring that a safe exit plan is always available. Address the patient calmly and attempt to understand the patient's motivations and needs. Providing for the patient's physical needs may enable you to start building rapport with the patient, calming his/her fears and reflexively aggressive behaviors. Generous listening may allow the patient to feel heard and appreciated, and lead to better communication throughout the visit.

If verbal management is ineffective, then it is appropriate to move to pharmacologic interventions. If the patient is willing and able, first offer oral medications. If the patient is unwilling to comply with this plan, it may be necessary to administer intravenous or intramuscular medications. Administration of these medications should only be attempted if it can be accomplished without compromising staff safety. This decision will be individualized depending on the patient's presentation and the resources available at the site. If medication cannot be safely administered and the patient is posing a risk to self or others, then a plan should be made to proceed with physical restraints. After application, it may be necessary to administer chemical restraint as well, once medical staff can safely perform these actions.

The decision to physically restrain a patient is a difficult one. This action impinges on a patient's civil rights and liberties by removing the ability to refuse care, freedom to associate, and freedom from imprisonment. This must be balanced against the need to protect healthcare workers from bodily harm, as well as the need to identify and treat possible emergent conditions that may be contributing to the patient's violent presentation. If the balance of this decision tips toward restraint, a coordinated plan should be created among all ED staff to ensure that everyone agrees and is aware of the intended course of action.

Methods of Physical Restraint

Methods for applying safe and effective physical restraints should focus on shielding the healthcare team from harm, as well as preventing patients from harming themselves. While restraint application represents a period of high risk to personnel, physicians should not be lulled into a false sense of security after application is completed. Patients may find way to hit, kick, spit, or otherwise inflict harm even while restrained. Furthermore, patients may be able to harm themselves while restrained, whether by struggling against restraints, twisting around the fixed points of a restraint, or flipping over their gurney by rocking or thrashing.

Best practice for applying physical restraints suggests that if limbs are to be restrained, all four limbs should initially be restrained. Patients are at increased risk for a twisting or flipping injury if only one or two limbs are restrained. Strategies for leg restraints may including securing the restraint to opposite corners of the bed (i.e., right leg to left corner, left leg to right corner), which will decrease the patient's ability to kick out toward health-care providers. Arm restraints may be used in an up/down fashion, as this limits the patient's ability to create momentum from rocking that might be used to flip a gurney. All restraints should be secured to the bed frame itself and never to bed rails, which are potentially mobile.

Patient positioning is important to reduce risk. Patients should always be supine, as prone or "hogtie" positioning increases suffocation risk. To further decrease this risk, pillows should also be removed. The head of the bed should be elevated to 30 degrees to decrease risk of aspiration. Care should be taken to minimize pressure points, and nursing staff should employ standard patient positioning tactics to decrease risk of pressure ulcers, especially if the patient is later chemically sedated.

Complications of Physical Restraint Use

The use of physical restraints is directly linked to multiple medical complications. Common complications include dehydration due to lack of ability to freely consume liquids and pressure-related skin breakdown due to lack of freedom of movement. Appropriate positioning and application of restraints can help to limit complications such as aspiration and limb ischemia. Serious, rare complications, including thromboembolic events, fractures, stress cardiomyopathy, asphyxia, and death, have been reported.

In addition to the medical risks of restraints, the cognitive biases introduced by the need for restraint application may cause physicians to miss a potentially life-threatening underlying diagnosis that is contributing to the patient's violent presentation. Standard medical workup, including point-of-care and laboratory testing, may be delayed if obtaining blood is dangerous for medical staff members. Imaging may be delayed or may be obtained in a suboptimal manner, leading to missed or delayed diagnoses. A detailed history and physical exam may be limited in these circumstances, which may impair the physician's ability to provide a complete and accurate assessment of a patient's condition, leading to adverse consequences.

The psychological effects of being physically restrained should not be overlooked. Surveys of patients who were restrained highlight a substantial loss of trust in the medical community, which may limit the patient's willingness to seek care in the future for medical or psychiatric illness. To mitigate this risk, physicians should thoroughly communicate with patients about the restraint process and give clear information about the process for gaining freedom of movement or removal of restraints in a timely manner. Even if you are unsure of a patient's ability to hear or understand information, every effort should still be made to verbally explain the processes in place.

Monitoring, Documentation, and Discontinuation of Restraints

To reduce these risks of physical restraints, the healthcare team should monitor the patient frequently during this critical period. The team should monitor vital signs, make neurovascular checks of each restrained extremity distal to the level of restraint to ensure adequate perfusion, and perform regular changes in positioning to prevent pressure injury. These measures must be implemented as well as carefully documented according to your local policy. Documentation should include the reasons for the application of physical restraints, the time and method of restraint, the results of continuous monitoring efforts, and the reasons for continuing restraint or for discontinuation.

Discontinuation of restraints should be attempted as soon as possible to reduce the risk of complications. Once the patient is calm and demonstrates his/her ability to cooperate with the healthcare team, restraints can be removed one limb at a time, giving the patient increasing opportunities for freedom of movement. Once all restraints have been removed, the patient should have continued close observation with a specific plan in place should the situation begin to escalate again.

CASE RESOLUTION

Due to the immediate threat to medical staff and failure of verbal de-escalation, you place the patient in physical restraints. Soft restraints are placed on all four extremities and secured to the bed frame, using an up/down configuration for the upper extremities and tying each leg to the opposite corner. After the patient is secure, intramuscular medications are given. The patient is placed on a pulse oximeter, cardiac monitoring is initiated, and nursing staff begins frequent neurovascular checks of the restrained extremities. The patient becomes more calm and is able to participate in an interview, in which you explain the need for restraints as well as the criteria for their removal. After demonstrating ability to comply with staff instructions and agreeing to oral antipsychotic medications, restraints are removed in a stepwise fashion. The patient has an appropriate medical workup, including evaluation by a psychiatrist, and he is ultimately admitted to an inpatient facility for further psychiatric stabilization.

KEY POINTS TO REMEMBER

- If staff safety allows, attempt verbal de-escalation and pharmacologic interventions before using physical restraints.
- If used, physical restraints should be applied to all four extremities with the patient in a supine, semi-upright position.
- Frequent monitoring, including cardiovascular monitoring and monitoring of restrained extremities, is crucial to ensure patient safety.

Further Reading

American College of Emergency Physicians (ACEP). Use of patient restraints: Policy statement. *Ann Emerg Med.* 2014;64(5):574.

Coburn VA, Mycyk MG. Physical and chemical restraints. *Emerg Med Clin North Am.* 2009;27(4):655–667.

Mason J, Colwell CB, Grock A. Agitation crisis control. *Ann Emerg Med*. 2019;72(4):371–373.

Miner JR, Klein LR, Cole JB, et al. The characteristics and prevalence of agitation in an urban county emergency department. *Ann Emerg Med*. 2018;72:361–370.

Wong AH, Crispino L, Parker JB, et al. Characteristics and severity of agitation associated with use of sedatives and restraints in the emergency department. *J Emerg Med*. 2019;57(5):611–619.

6   The SAFE-T Wasn't On

Bruce J. Grattan Jr.

A 73-year-old man presents to your ED after his neighbor called EMS when the patient "was acting strange." On presentation, the patient is somnolent and appears malnourished. His Glasgow Coma Scale (GCS) score is 13 for confusion and eye opening. He smells of alcohol, is slow to respond, and does not make eye contact. He has poor hygiene and a flat affect. There are burns to his right hand, as well as to his face and neck on the right side, with associated scattered abrasions and swelling. His right forearm has an open wound with minimal bleeding. When asked what happened, he says, "It was nothing, just an accident. I must have slipped working on something." He repeatedly asks to be left alone so he can go home. Past medical history is significant for alcohol abuse and chronic pain from injuries sustained in the Marine Corps. Vitals are BP 185/93, HR 93, RR 12, SpO_2 96% on room air, temp 36.9°C.

What do you do now?

THE SUICIDAL PATIENT

Background

Globally, suicide takes a life every 40 seconds.[1] It is the fourth leading cause of death in the United States among those aged 35 to 54 and the 10th leading cause of death overall,[2] and rates are increasing dramatically.[3] There are nearly 650,000 ED evaluations for suicide attempts annually.[4] Suicide and self-harm are estimated to cost $70 billion annually.[5]

Regardless of chief complaint, nearly 10% of all adult patients presenting to the ED have been shown to have recent suicidal ideation or behavior, and currently the Joint Commission requires screening for suicidal ideation for all patients presenting to the ED. Such screening has been shown to be effective and does not appear to negatively affect ED throughput.

Patient Safety

The safety of the patient and staff must take priority. Patients should be searched for weapons and direct and continuous patient monitoring should be initiated. The patient's surroundings in the ED should be assessed and risk of harm minimized, which may necessitate removal of needles, tubing, and other potential hazards. Ideally, a separate behavioral health unit/area of the department should be used when available. Once safety is ensured, assess the airway, breathing, and circulatory status, being particularly mindful of evidence of toxidromes or injuries. A full medical exam is indicated in the presence of abnormal vital signs or based upon the history and review of systems.

Mental Status Evaluation

When eliciting a history from a suicidal patient it is vital to use a non-judgmental tone and accurately identify the extent of any injuries and ingestions. Use open-ended questions while maintaining an empathetic and direct approach. Goals of the history are to determine how much and at what time any ingestion occurred and to elicit whether the patient has an ongoing intent of self-harm. To this end, it is often necessary to gather collateral history from any family, friends, or EMS personnel, as the patient may not be able or willing to divulge the details of what took place.

The focused psychiatric assessment can be remembered using the mnemonic "Depressed Patients Seem Anxious, So Claim Psychiatrists":

- **D**epression and mood disorders (major depression, bipolar disorder, dysthymia)
- **P**ersonality disorders (borderline personality disorder)
- **S**ubstance abuse disorders
- **A**nxiety disorders (panic disorder, obsessive-compulsive disorder)
- **S**omatization disorder and eating disorders
- **C**ognitive disorders (dementia, delirium)
- **P**sychotic disorders (schizophrenia, delusional disorder and psychosis accompanying depression, substance abuse or dementia)

Risk Factors

A number of suicide risk factors have been identified, including depression, physical illness, relationship difficulties, low socioeconomic status, and alcohol abuse. Putting this in perspective, a recent meta-analysis calculated odds ratios (ORs) for various risk factors. Risk factors for suicidal ideation included prior suicidal ideation (OR 3.55), hopelessness (OR 3.28), and depression (OR 2.45). Risk factors for suicide attempts included prior non-suicidal self-injury (OR 4.15), prior suicide attempt (OR 3.41), and prior hospitalization (OR 2.32). Prior psychiatric hospitalization and prior suicide attempt were the strongest risk factors for suicide death, with ORs of 3.57 and 2.24, respectively.[6]

Suicide risk is greatest after diagnosis of any mental disorder, and patients with prior psychiatric admission are also at much greater lifetime risk compared with the general population (8.6% vs. 0.5%). Depression is a well-recognized risk factor for suicide, and approximately 10% of depressed adults will die by suicide. Women attempt suicide four times more often than men, yet suicide attempts in men are three times more lethal. Those patients who have made a previous suicide attempts are six times more likely to make another attempt. Alcohol abuse is a major risk factor for suicide completion, and it is not uncommon for patients to present to the ED with both suicidal ideation and alcohol intoxication. This can be a complicated scenario as patients may transiently express suicidal ideation that resolves when sober. A conservative approach to this situation is warranted, and it is best to observe the patient and refrain from a suicide risk assessment until the patient is no longer intoxicated. There is no evidence that directly asking about suicide increases a patient's risk.

Screening Tools

Assessing suicidality is challenging, as nearly 80% of those who die by suicide deny suicidal thoughts just prior to death. Despite national guidelines recommending risk assessment, there is no current standard of care. There are several screening tools available, including the Suicide Assessment and Five-Step Evaluation and Triage (SAFE-T) tool,[7] the Sheehan Suicidality Tracking Scale (S-STS),[8] the Columbia Suicide Severity Rating Scale (C-SSRS),[9], and the ICAR^{2}E tool.[10]

The SAFE-T tool assesses internal and external protective factors and coping skills and the presence/absence of suicidal plan, intent, and history of suicidal behavior to attempt to aid clinical decision-making.[11] The S-STS is the only tool that has been shown to be predictive of further suicide attempts within the next 6 months and recently was validated in an ED population in South Korea; however, the external validity of this study may be limited.

Distinguishing between planned and unplanned suicide attempts can be helpful in risk stratification as planned attempts are more often lethal and associated with greater severity of depressive symptoms. The C-SSRS uses previously identified factors that have been found to be predictive of both suicide attempt and completion. This tool helps separate suicidal ideation from suicidal behavior. The C-SSRS assesses several subdomains, including lethality, suicide behavior, intensity, and ideation[12] (Figure 6.1).

Through a collaboration between the American College of Emergency Physicians (ACEP) and the American Foundation for Suicide Prevention, a working group was established to develop a simple evidence-based mnemonic for ED providers. Based on the results of both an expert census panel and a systematic literature review, the ICAR^{2}E tool was developed. It has been published by ACEP, is free and available online (https://www.acep.org/iCar2e), and can be a useful reference with printable brochures and other materials. This tool serves as a mnemonic outlining the steps taken for suicide screening: *I*dentify suicide risk, *C*ommunicate, *A*ssess for life threats

Step 1: Identify Risk Factors	
C-SSRS Suicidal Ideation Severity	**Month**
1) Wish to be dead *Have you wished you were dead or wished you could go to sleep and not wake up?*	
2) Current suicidal thoughts *Have you actually had any thoughts of killing yourself?*	
3) Suicidal thoughts w/ Method (w/no specific Plan or Intent or act) *Have you been thinking about how you might do this?*	
4) Suicidal Intent without Specific Plan *Have you had these thoughts and had some intention of acting on them?*	
5) Intent with Plan *Have you started to work out or worked out the details of how to kill yourself?* *Do you intend to carry out this plan?*	

C-SSRS Suicidal Behavior: *"Have you ever done anything, started to do anything, or prepared to do anything to end your life?"*	**Lifetime**
Examples: Collected pills, obtained a gun, gave away valuables, wrote a will or suicide note, took out pills but didn't swallow any, held a gun but changed your mind or it was grabbed from your hand, went to the roof but didn't jump; or actually took pills, tried to shoot yourself, cut yourself, tried to hang yourself, etc. If "YES" Was it within the past 3 months?	**Past 3 Months**

Activating Events:
- ☐ Recent losses or other significant negative event(s) (legal, financial, relationship, etc.)
- ☐ Pending incarceration or homelessness
- ☐ Current or pending isolation or feeling alone

Treatment History:
- ☐ Previous psychiatric diagnosis and treatments
- ☐ Hopeless or dissatisfied with treatment
- ☐ Non-compliant with treatment
- ☐ Not receiving treatment
- ☐ Insomnia

Other:
- ☐ _____
- ☐ _____
- ☐ _____

Clinical Status:
- ☐ Hopelessness
- ☐ Major depressive episode
- ☐ Mixed affect episode (e.g. Bipolar)
- ☐ Command Hallucinations to hurt self
- ☐ Chronic physical pain or other acute medical problem (e.g. CNS disorders)
- ☐ Highly impulsive behavior
- ☐ Substance abuse or dependence
- ☐ Agitation or severe anxiety
- ☐ Perceived burden on family or others
- ☐ Homicidal Ideation
- ☐ Aggressive behavior towards others
- ☐ Refuses or feels unable to agree to safety plan
- ☐ Sexual abuse (lifetime)
- ☐ Family history of suicide

☐ **Access to lethal methods:** Ask specifically about presence or absence of a firearm in the home or ease of accessing

Step 2: Identify Protective Factors (Protective factors may not counteract significant acute suicide risk factors)

Internal:
- ☐ Fear of death or dying due to pain and suffering
- ☐ Identifies reasons for living
- ☐ _____
- ☐ _____

External:
- ☐ Belief that suicide is immoral; high spirituality
- ☐ Responsibility to family or others; living with family
- ☐ Supportive social network of family or friends
- ☐ Engaged in work or school

FIGURE 6.1 SAFE-T with C-SSRS

Source: https://cssrs.columbia.edu/about-the-project/about-the-lighthouse-project/

Step 3: Specific questioning about Thoughts, Plans, and Suicidal Intent – (see Step 1 for Ideation Severity and Behavior)	
C-SSRS Suicidal Ideation Intensity (with respect to the most severe ideation 1-5 identified above)	**Month**
Frequency *How many times have you had these thoughts?* (1) Less than once a week (2) Once a week (3) 2-5 times in week (4) Daily or almost daily (5) Many times each day	
Duration *When you have the thoughts how long do they last?* (1) Fleeting - few seconds or minutes (4) 4-8 hours/most of day (2) Less than 1 hour/some of the time (5) More than 8 hours/persistent or continuous (3) 1-4 hours/a lot of time	
Controllability *Could/can you stop thinking about killing yourself or wanting to die if you want to?* (1) Easily able to control thoughts (4) Can control thoughts with a lot of difficulty (2) Can control thoughts with little difficulty (5) Unable to control thoughts (3) Can control thoughts with some difficulty (0) Does not attempt to control thoughts	
Deterrents *Are there things - anyone or anything (e.g., family, religion, pain of death) - that stopped you from wanting to die or acting on thoughts of suicide?* (1) Deterrents definitely stopped you from attempting suicide (4) Deterrents most likely did not stop you (2) Deterrents probably stopped you (5) Deterrents definitely did not stop you (3) Uncertain that deterrents stopped you (0) Does not apply	
Reasons for Ideation *What sort of reasons did you have for thinking about wanting to die or killing yourself? Was it to end the pain or stop the way you were feeling (in other words you couldn't go on living with this pain or how you were feeling) or was it to get attention, revenge or a reaction from others? Or both?* (1) Completely to get attention, revenge or a reaction from others (4) Mostly to end or stop the pain (you couldn't go on living with the pain or how you were feeling) (2) Mostly to get attention, revenge or reaction from others (5) Completely to end or stop the pain (you couldn't go on living with the pain or how you were feeling) (3) Equally to get attention, revenge or a reaction from others and to end/stop the pain (0) Does not apply	
Total Score	

FIGURE 6.1 Continued

Step 4: Guidelines to Determine Level of Risk and Develop Interventions to LOWER Risk Level

"The estimation of suicide risk, at the culmination of the suicide assessment, is the quintessential **clinical judgment**, since no study has identified one specific risk factor or set of risk factors as specifically predictive of suicide or other suicidal behavior."

From The American Psychiatric Association Practice Guidelines for the Assessment and Treatment of Patients with Suicidal Behaviors, page 24.

RISK STRATIFICATION	TRIAGE
High Suicide Risk ☐ Suicidal ideation with intent or intent with plan in past month (C-SSRS Suicidal Ideation #4 or #5) Or ☐ Suicidal behavior within past 3 months (C-SSRS Suicidal Behavior)	☐ Initiate local psychiatric admission process ☐ Stay with patient until transfer to higher level of care is complete ☐ Follow-up and document outcome of emergency psychiatric evaluation
Moderate Suicide Risk ☐ Suicidal ideation with method, **WITHOUT plan, intent or behavior** in past month (C-SSRS Suicidal Ideation #3) Or ☐ Suicidal behavior more than 3 months ago (C-SSRS Suicidal Behavior Lifetime) Or ☐ Multiple risk factors and few protective factors	☐ Directly address suicide risk, implementing suicide prevention strategies ☐ Develop Safety Plan
Low Suicide Risk ☐ Wish to die or Suicidal Ideation **WITHOUT method, intent, plan or behavior** (C-SSRS Suicidal Ideation #1 or #2) Or ☐ Modifiable risk factors and strong protective factors Or ☐ No reported history of Suicidal Ideation or Behavior	☐ Discretionary Outpatient Referral

Step 5: Documentation

Risk Level :

[ ] High Suicide Risk
[ ] Moderate Suicide Risk
[ ] Low Suicide Risk

Clinical Note:

☐ Your Clinical Observation
☐ Relevant Mental Status Information
☐ Methods of Suicide Risk Evaluation

☐ Brief Evaluation Summary
  ☐ Warning Signs
  ☐ Risk Indicators
  ☐ Protective Factors
  ☐ Access to Lethal Means
  ☐ Collateral Sources Used and Relevant Information Obtained
  ☐ Specific Assessment Data to Support Risk Determination
  ☐ Rationale for Actions Taken and Not Taken

☐ Provision of Crisis Line 1-800-273-TALK(8255)
☐ Implementation of Safety Plan (If Applicable)

FIGURE 6.1 Continued

and ensure safety, *R*isk assessment, *R*educe the risk, *E*xtend care beyond the *E*mergency department visit.

However, none of these tools have been validated for determination of patient disposition or risk stratification. Regardless of the screening tools used, the effects of even a single risk assessment in the ED are profound, with evidence suggesting upward of a 40% short-term risk reduction of suicidal behavior.[13]

Disposition and Planning for Safety/Lethal Means Counseling

For patients in the ED with suicidal gestures, the risk of repeat suicide attempt is upward of 25%. Among those presenting to the ED with self-harm, rates of any form of repeat self-harm are upward of 27% within 6 months. Safety planning involves an individualized step-by-step guide formulated through an individualized collaboration with the patient to help those at risk for suicide to identify warning signs of a return of suicidality and address them proactively. This is an important and often overlooked step. Safety planning has been shown to reduce subsequent suicide attempts by 30% to 50%[14,15] and is endorsed as a best practice by the Suicide Prevention Resource Center.[7] As part of safety planning, physicians should conduct *lethal means counseling*, an evidence-based strategy to reduce both suicide attempts and death. Lethal means counseling identifies the patient's access to items such as firearms that could be used for self-harm.[16,17] *Safety planning* should consist of an individualized, prioritized written list of coping strategies that the patient can use to offset a crisis, such as contacting supporting resources and implementing internal coping strategies.

Even when low-risk patients are discharged, it is vital to have appropriate follow-up. Evidence suggests that email/mail contacts, brief telephone contacts, or other "caring contacts," even if automated, reduce both suicide attempts and death. Those working in EDs with limited resources should be aware that low-risk patients do not require an emergency mental health consultation.

CASE RESOLUTION

After clinical sobriety and with additional history corroborated by the patient's neighbor, the ED physician learns that the patient had attempted suicide by placing a bullet in a vise and striking it with a hammer while trying to get his head in front of the projectile. He was distraught over the death of his wife 3 months earlier and had little/no social or family support. He had long suffered from untreated depression and posttraumatic stress disorder from his military service. His chronic pain provided him access to opiate medications. The bullet's casing lacerated his forearm, and he suffered powder burns and superficial soft tissue injury to his neck and face as a result of the explosion. Additionally, he was found to have taken a nonlethal overdose of his prescribed oxycodone prior to EMS arrival when his attempt failed. The patient initially experienced respiratory depression, which responded to naloxone. Once stable, he was monitored with suicide precautions and a 1:1 sitter. Imaging showed no retained foreign bodies or fractures, and his wounds were repaired. As part of lethal means counseling, he agreed to allow his firearms to be removed from his home. Given the severity of his attempt, he was admitted to inpatient psychiatric care.

KEY POINTS TO REMEMBER

- Know risk factors as well as protective factors.
- Elderly males with access to firearms are at high risk.
- Even low-risk patients who are discharged need follow-up.
- Involve family and friends both for information regarding the event and safety at discharge.
- Prepare a safety plan: Have a written agreement of what steps the patient will take when experiencing suicidal thoughts, including how to identify warning signs and develop coping strategies.
- Familiarize yourself with screening tools, but recognize their limitations.

References

1. WHO. Preventing suicide: A global imperative. 2014. https://apps.who.int/iris/bitstream/handle/10665/131056/9789241564779_eng.pdf?sequence=1
2. Centers for Disease Control and Prevention. Ten leading causes of death and injury. CDC Injury Prevention and Control. https://www.cdc.gov/injury/wisqars/LeadingCauses.html

3. Curtin S, Heron M. Death rates due to suicide and homicide among persons aged 10–24: United States, 2000–2017. Centers for Disease Control and Prevention. https://www.cdc.gov/nchs/data/databriefs/db352-h.pdf

4. Canner JK, Giuliano K, Selvarajah S, et al. Emergency department visits for attempted suicide and self harm in the USA: 2006–2013. *Epidemiol Psychiatr Sci.* 2018;27(1):94–102.

5. Centers for Disease Control and Prevention. Suicide fast facts. 2019. https://www.cdc.gov/violenceprevention/suicide/fastfact.html?CDC_AA_refVal=https%3A%2F%2Fwww.cdc.gov%2Fviolenceprevention%2Fsuicide%2Fconsequences.html

6. Franklin JC, Ribeiro JD, Fox KR, et al. Risk factors for suicidal thoughts and behaviors: A meta-analysis of 50 years of research. *Psychol Bull.* 2017;143(2):187–232.

7. Suicide Prevention Resource Center. Caring for adult patients with suicide risk: A consensus-based guide for emergency departments. https://www.sprc.org/edguide

8. Coric V, Stock EG, Pultz J, et al. Sheehan Suicidality Tracking Scale (Sheehan-STS): Preliminary results from a multicenter clinical trial in generalized anxiety disorder. *Psychiatry.* 2009;6(1):26–31.

9. Lindh AU, Waern M, Beckman K, et al. Short-term risk of non-fatal and fatal suicidal behaviours: The predictive validity of the Columbia-Suicide Severity Rating Scale in a Swedish adult psychiatric population with a recent episode of self-harm. *BMC Psychiatry.* 2018;18(1):319.

10. American College of Emergency Physicians. ICAR²E: A tool for managing suicidal patients in the ED. 2020. https://www.acep.org/patient-care/iCar2e/

11. Jacobs D. *Screening for Mental Health: A Resource Guide for Implementing the Joint Commission 2007 Patient Safety Goals on Suicide.* Wellesley Hills, MA: Screening for Mental Health, Inc.; 2007.

12. Posner K, Brown GK, Stanley B, et al. The Columbia-Suicide Severity Rating Scale: Initial validity and internal consistency findings from three multisite studies with adolescents and adults. *Am J Psychiatry.* 2011;168(12):1266–1277.

13. Kapur N, Steeg S, Webb R, et al. Does clinical management improve outcomes following self-harm? Results from the multicentre study of self-harm in England. *PLoS One.* 2013;8(8):e70434.

14. Miller IW, Camargo CA, Jr., Arias SA, et al. Suicide prevention in an emergency department population: The ED-SAFE study. *JAMA Psychiatry.* 2017;74(6):563–570.

15. Stanley B, Brown GK, Brenner LA, et al. Comparison of the safety planning intervention with follow-up vs. usual care of suicidal patients treated in the emergency department. *JAMA Psychiatry.* 2018;75(9):894–900.

16. Barber CW, Miller MJ. Reducing a suicidal person's access to lethal means of suicide: A research agenda. *Am J Prev Med.* 2014;47(3 Suppl 2):S264–S272.

17. Suicide Prevention Resource Center. Suicide prevention fact sheets. 2019. https://www.sprc.org/resources-programs

7 Risky Business

Jillian L. McGrath and Lydia M. Sahlani

A 53-year-old White male presents to the ED complaining of feeling depressed. He reports feeling down and hopeless for several months after losing his job. He has a remote history of major depression and took antidepressant medication in the past. He denies other medical problems or current medications. He is single and lives alone. He denies auditory, visual, or command hallucinations. He reports poor appetite and sleep. He drinks six or seven beers daily and denies any history of withdrawal symptoms. He denies illicit drug use. When asked, he discloses that he has had suicidal thoughts for the past few weeks and has considered several possible plans. He reports fatigue, but review of systems is otherwise negative. His vital signs are normal. His affect is flat and responses are slow, but the remaining physical exam is unremarkable. He initially agrees to remain in the ED for evaluation by your psychiatric consultant, but his nurse later tells you that the patient is tired of waiting and is requesting to be discharged.

What do you do now?

ASSESSING SUICIDE RISK

It is imperative that patients presenting to the ED with complaints of suicidal ideation or thoughts of self-harm are appropriately assessed for suicide risk. Suicide is a growing public health concern and is the 10th leading cause of death in the United States, resulting in more than 48,000 deaths in 2018.[1] Suicide affects patients of all ages. It is the second leading cause of death for people 10 to 34 years of age, the fourth leading cause among people 35 to 54 years of age, and the eighth leading cause among people 55 to 64 years of age.[1] ED physicians and other providers must be aware of the long-term risk factors for suicide and recognize acute crisis scenarios so they can develop a safe plan for disposition. In this case, the provider must carefully assess the patient's risk for suicide to determine whether the patient is safe to be discharged at his request. If it is determined that he is an imminent risk to himself, then appropriate suicide precautions are indicated. These precautions may include involuntary hold orders as well as physical and chemical restraint.[2]

This case highlights several patient characteristics that correlate with long-term risk of suicide. First, the patient's demographics predict higher suicide risk:

- Race: White and Native American patients have the highest overall suicide rates.
- Gender: Males are three to four times more likely to die by suicide (due to more frequent use of lethal means) than females. White men account for the majority of suicide deaths in the older population.[1]
- Past medical history: The patient has a history of mood disorder (major depression) that is not currently managed with medication or outpatient psychiatric care. Other disorders that can increase long-term risk include chronic medical illness or other psychiatric conditions such as schizophrenia, anxiety, posttraumatic stress disorder, or personality disorders. This patient's history of substance abuse further increases his risk for suicide. His history is also suggestive of social isolation and poor social support; thus, he lacks protective factors that mitigate risk.

Many other important factors, not specific to this case, should be considered when assessing risk. Some examples are social considerations such as patients identifying as lesbian, gay, bisexual, and transgender or those who belong to groups where a cultural or social stigma around mental health diagnosis and treatment exists.

Patients often present to the ED during an acute crisis. The acute stressor of loss of employment may be considered a trigger or precipitating event for this patient. Other stressors that may precipitate an acute crisis include significant professional or financial losses or social stressors such as deaths or difficult relationships. There are details about the patient in this case that should prompt further inquiry by the treating provider. Inquiring about past suicidal behavior or attempts is important as their presence may increase his long-term risk (although many suicide victims have no known history or prior attempts). One must also consider his specific plan(s) and assess whether they involve potentially lethal means. Access to weapons or firearms increases suicide risk.

DECISION TOOLS

Following a focused medical assessment, an objective decision tool should be used to help identify suicide risk. A brief assessment of suicide risk should be performed for this patient after his clinical sobriety and decision-making capacity are confirmed. For a patient who is determined to be at a low suicide risk based on a brief assessment, a safety plan and outpatient management may be appropriate. However, this patient's current suicidal ideation, history of mental illness, and substance abuse exclude him from a low-risk category appropriate for outpatient management. Therefore, a more comprehensive assessment of suicide risk should be completed and/or psychiatric consultation should be obtained. This may include psychiatric consultation or application of the Suicide Assessment and Five-Step Evaluation and Triage (SAFE-T) protocol (Figure 7.1). SAFE-T, an example of a comprehensive suicide assessment protocol, guides clinicians through five steps that address the patient's level of suicide risk and then suggests appropriate interventions. The steps are as follows:

1. Identify risk factors.
2. Identify protective factors.

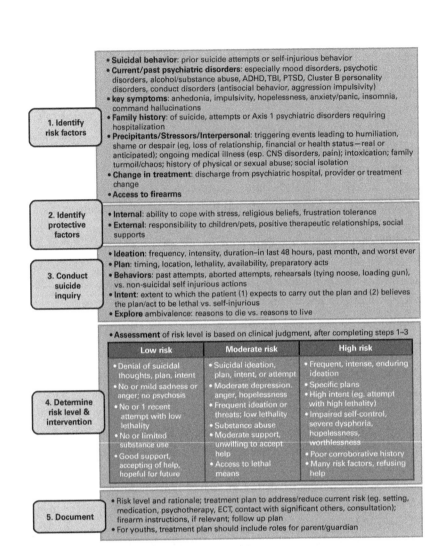

1. Identify risk factors
- **Suicidal behavior:** prior suicide attempts or self-injurious behavior
- **Current/past psychiatric disorders:** especially mood disorders, psychotic disorders, alcohol/substance abuse, ADHD, TBI, PTSD, Cluster B personality disorders, conduct disorders (antisocial behavior, aggression impulsivity)
- **key symptoms:** anhedonia, impulsivity, hopelessness, anxiety/panic, insomnia, command hallucinations
- **Family history:** of suicide, attempts or Axis 1 psychiatric disorders requiring hospitalization
- **Precipitants/Stressors/Interpersonal:** triggering events leading to humiliation, shame or despair (eg, loss of relationship, financial or health status—real or anticipated); ongoing medical illness (esp. CNS disorders, pain); intoxication; family turmoil/chaos; history of physical or sexual abuse; social isolation
- **Change in treatment:** discharge from psychiatric hospital, provider or treatment change
- **Access to firearms**

2. Identify protective factors
- **Internal:** ability to cope with stress, religious beliefs, frustration tolerance
- **External:** responsibility to children/pets, positive therapeutic relationships, social supports

3. Conduct suicide inquiry
- **Ideation:** frequency, intensity, duration–in last 48 hours, past month, and worst ever
- **Plan:** timing, location, lethality, availability, preparatory acts
- **Behaviors:** past attempts, aborted attempts, rehearsals (tying noose, loading gun), vs. non-suicidal self injurious actions
- **Intent:** extent to which the patient (1) expects to carry out the plan and (2) believes the plan/act to be lethal vs. self-injurious
- **Explore** ambivalence: reasons to die vs. reasons to live

4. Determine risk level & intervention
- **Assessment** of risk level is based on clinical judgment, after completing steps 1–3

Low risk	Moderate risk	High risk
• Denial of suicidal thoughts, plan, intent	• Suicidal ideation, plan, intent, or attempt	• Frequent, intense, enduring ideation
• No or mild sadness or anger; no psychosis	• Moderate depression, anger, hopelessness	• Specific plans
• No or 1 recent attempt with low lethality	• Frequent ideation or threats; low lethality	• High intent (eg. attempt with high lethality)
• No or limited substance use	• Substance abuse	• Impaired self-control, severe dysphoria, hopelessness, worthlessness
• Good support, accepting of help, hopeful for future	• Moderate support, unwilling to accept help	• Poor corroborative history
	• Access to lethal means	• Many risk factors, refusing help

5. Document
- Risk level and rationale; treatment plan to address/reduce current risk (eg. setting, medication, psychotherapy, ECT, contact with significant others, consultation); firearm instructions, if relevant; follow up plan
- For youths, treatment plan should include roles for parent/guardian

FIGURE 7.1 Suicide Assessment Five-Step Evaluation and Triage (SAFE-T) protocol

Betz, Marian E., Rosen's Emergency Medicine: Concepts and Clinical Practice, Chapter 105, 1366–1373.e3 Suicide assessment five-step evaluation and triage. (Modified from Davidson CL, Olson-Madden JH, Betz ME, et al: Emergency department identification, assessment, and management of the suicidal patient. In Koslow SH, Ruiz P, Nemeroff CB, editors: A concise guide to understanding suicide. United Kingdom, 2014, Cambridge University Press, pp 244–255; Suicide Assessment Five-Step Evaluation and Triage [SAFE-T]. Substance Abuse and Mental Health Services Administration. http://store.samhsa.gov.proxy.lib.ohio-state.edu/product/Suicide-Assessment-Five-Step-Evaluation-and-Triage-SAFE-T-/SMA09-4432

3. Conduct suicide inquiry
4. Determine risk level/intervention.
5. Document.[3]

Other similar tools may be used to risk stratify patients and develop a therapeutic plan.

CASE RESOLUTION

In this case, it would be prudent to have an empathetic discussion with the patient detailing concern for his safety. Ideally, he would agree to a voluntary assessment by your psychiatry consultant. Based on the risk factors discussed earlier, this patient would be considered to be at least moderate risk for suicide. Should the patient decline voluntary evaluation, placing an involuntary hold would be appropriate to ensure adequate psychiatric intervention and to avoid imminent danger to the patient.

KEY POINTS TO REMEMBER

- Suicide affects patients of all ages and is a leading cause of death in the United States.
- Many vulnerable groups exist, including adolescents, older adults, White or Native American persons, or those who identify as LGBTQ.
- Long-term risk is increased for patients with a history of mood disorders, substance disorders, or prior suicidal behavior.
- Acute crises may trigger suicide, including professional, financial, and social stressors.
- Access to weapons, firearms, or other lethal means increases suicide risk.
- A brief assessment should be employed by ED physicians and providers to identify patients who require more comprehensive evaluation or psychiatric consultation.

References

1. Centers for Disease Control and Prevention. Web-Based Injury Statistics Query and Reporting System (WISQARS). 2020. https://www.cdc.gov/injury/wisqars/index.html
2. Betz ME, Caterino JM. Suicide. In: Walls R, Hockberger R, Gausche-Hill M, eds. *Rosen's Emergency Medicine: Concepts and Clinical Practice*. 9th ed. Philadelphia: Elsevier; 2018:1366–1373.
3. Substance Abuse and Mental Health Services Administration. Suicide Assessment Five-Step Evaluation and Triage (SAFE-T) pocket card. 2009. http://store.samhsa.gov/product/Suicide-Assessment-Five-Step-Evaluation-and-Triage-SAFE-T-/SMA09-4432

Further Reading

Betz ME, Boudreaux ED. Managing suicidal patients in the emergency department. *Ann Emerg Med*. 2016;67(2):276–282. doi:10.1016/j.annemergmed.2015.09.001

Betz ME, Caterino JM. Suicide. In: Walls R, Hockberger R, Gausche-Hill M, eds. *Rosen's Emergency Medicine: Concepts and Clinical Practice*. 9th ed. Philadelphia: Elsevier; 2018:1366–1373.

Colpe LJ, Pringle BA. Data for building a national suicide prevention strategy: What we have and what we need. *Am J Prev Med*. 2014;47:S130–S136.

Rodgers P. Understanding risk and protective factors for suicide: A primer for preventing suicide. Suicide Prevention Resource Center. 2019. https://www.sprc.org/resources-programs/understanding-risk-protective-factors-suicide-primer-preventing-suicide

Suicide Prevention Resource Center. Caring for adult patients with suicide risk: A consensus-based guide for emergency departments. https://www.sprc.org/edguide

8 Danger in the Mirror

Max Hensel and Carmen Wolfe

A 32-year-old male is brought in by ambulance for evaluation of a laceration. EMS personnel report that they were called to the scene by bystanders who found the patient sitting on a bench with blood streaming down his arms. They note that the patient seemed withdrawn and was unwilling to give them any information about his injury. On examination they noted deep lacerations over his left upper extremity with bleeding controlled by a pressure dressing and not requiring placement of a tourniquet. Upon initial evaluation of the patient, you find him to be awake and alert, though reticent to speak with you. HR is 106 and BP is 132/78. You remove the blood-soaked bandage from his left forearm, revealing a linear laceration that is now hemostatic. In addition to his current injury, you also note multiple healed scars on bilateral upper extremities. The patient continues to state, "I don't know how this happened again."

What do you do now?

SELF-HARM IN THE PSYCHIATRIC PATIENT

Self-harm, also known as non-suicidal self-injury (NSSI), is a broad term encompassing a multitude of self-inflicted behaviors intended to destroy bodily tissue. As opposed to suicidal behavior, the term *self-harm* indicates a lack of intention to die, though these behaviors are associated with an increased risk of suicide attempts. Self-injurious behaviors may include typical presentations such as cutting, scratching, burning, hitting, self-amputation, ingestion of chemicals, or oral ingestion of dangerous foreign objects. Other more bizarre behaviors have been rarely reported, including ocular or genital self-mutilation.

INTERVIEWING A PATIENT WITH NSSI

NSSI is common, though only a small subset of patients will require emergent medical care for their injuries. Community samples of adolescents indicate that rates of NSSI may exceed 50%, with more than a quarter of those injuries being classified as moderate or severe. Understanding typical populations who are at risk for NSSI may help to guide appropriate interview techniques when patients present with self-harm injuries. Many psychiatric disorders, such as anxiety, depression, substance use disorders, and eating disorders, have all been correlated with NSSI. Patients who present in adolescence with self-harm injuries are more likely to develop psychiatric disorders later in life, so clinicians should use this opportunity to establish early referral for psychiatric services.

In the setting of concomitant psychiatric disease, obtaining a detailed history may be difficult. Patients may be withdrawn and unwilling to participate in the interview. Such an interaction can lead to frustration or anger on the part of the physician. Recognizing this negative countertransference allows the physician to acknowledge and set aside these feelings and move toward creating a therapeutic alliance with the patient to address both his/her medical and psychiatric needs.

It is important to ask direct questions related to the patient's intention of his/her self-harm as patients may not readily disclose information. Given that apparent NSSI is associated with increased risk for suicide attempts, it is important to maintain a high index of suspicion for possible suicidal intention. Approaching the patient with compassion, in a nonjudgmental fashion, will allow the physician to create a safe space for the patient to share his/her motivations for his/her behavior. Using alternative information sources such as EMS personnel, accompanying family members, or previous medical records is especially prudent in these cases to collect collateral information.

CUTTING INJURIES

The majority of self-harm injuries involve cutting with loss of skin integrity of varying degrees. A detailed physical exam is necessary to address all wounds as patients may conceal additional injuries. Location of wounds falls along gender lines, with women tending to inflict harm on the extremities, while men have an increased propensity to injure the face, chest, genitals, and hands. Most self-harm is superficial and does not warrant extensive medical intervention beyond basic wound care. Abrasions should be cleaned, dressed, and evaluated for signs of infection. Tetanus status should be known and updated if applicable. In the cases of lacerations, the same principles apply, with the additional goals of hemostasis and dermal repair. Initial evaluation should assess for signs of vascular injury, including active arterial bleeding. In this setting, a combination of direct pressure, direct vascular repair, or tourniquet use may be necessary to achieve hemostasis. Hemodynamic instability in the setting of active bleeding may require administration of blood products. After hemostasis is achieved, assessment of motor and sensory function of the distal extremity is necessary to ensure there are no associated nerve injuries. Following extensive irrigation and exploration of the wound for underlying structure damage, the wound should be closed with appropriate sutures and plans made for monitoring for infection and suture removal.

BURN INJURIES

Burns are approached by first determining scene safety for providers by assessing for need of decontamination. Patient may use a variety of agents to cause burns, such as caustic substances, cigarettes, lighters, or other household objects. Major burns may be associated with suicidal intent, with extreme cases, including self-immolation, being more common internationally and requiring immediate medical resuscitation. For minor burns, as is more often the case when associated with NSSI, the wound should be irrigated and pain control provided. Debridement should be provided if necessary, and partial- or full-thickness burns should be covered in a basic topical antibiotic with appropriate dressing. The type of burn as well as estimated total body surface area should be assessed; these findings will help determine if the patient meets criteria for transfer to a burn center. Attention should be given to the specific location of the burn. If burns are present on the face, eyes, ears, hands, perineum, or feet or involve major joints, the patient may require burn center referral.

DELIBERATE FOREIGN BODY INGESTION OR INSERTION

Patients may deliberately swallow a foreign body or may intentionally place a foreign body in an orifice, under the skin, or in a previous surgical incision site. The type of object inserted will help determine radiopacity and appropriate imaging options. For oral ingestions, the specific type and size of object will determine the safety to allow for natural passage rather than surgical retrieval. Objects such as button batteries, multiple magnets, or large objects may require surgical consultation and removal. In rare cases where patients place objects underneath the surface of their skin or in open surgical sites, it is important to choose appropriate imaging modalities, which may include plain radiographs, ultrasound, or CT. These injuries may have high infection rates and consideration should be given to prophylactic antibiotics. Superficial objects on the extremities may be able to be removed in the ED, but deeper foreign bodies or those in the face, abdomen, hands, or genitals may require consultation with specialty services.

INGESTION OF CAUSTIC OR PHARMACOLOGIC SUBSTANCES

Ingestion of caustic chemicals may cause significant damage to the GI tract as well as the larynx and tracheobronchial tree if aspirated. Alkali-induced injury, as is seen with ammonia and household cleaning products, causes primarily esophageal damage through liquefactive necrosis with possible penetrating injury. Acid-induced injury causes coagulative necrosis and is more highly associated with upper airway injuries and gastric injuries. Medical resuscitation and pain control are often required prior to psychiatric evaluation in these cases. Immediate complications may include aspiration, loss of airway control, esophageal perforation with mediastinitis, or gastric perforation with peritonitis. Delayed complications include bleeding, strictures, or more rarely fistulization.

Ingestion of pharmacologic substances such as prescription drugs, over-the-counter drugs, illicit drugs, or herbal substances can present in a variety of ways. Determination of type, dosage, and number of pills ingested will help guide evaluation, treatment, and appropriate observation period. Medical evaluation, including vital signs and a thorough physical exam, may point to a specific toxidrome. Consideration must be given to possible co-ingestants, with laboratory screening for acetaminophen overdose necessary given its asymptomatic initial presentation.

MAJOR SELF-MUTILATION

Examples of severe self-mutilation may be found in the literature in case reports and case series and typically involve ocular, genital, or extremity mutilation. In these rare instances, patients are more often reported to have a concomitant diagnosis of serious mental illness with psychosis present at the time of the event. Specific management addresses the medical emergency at hand, followed by immediate psychiatric evaluation. Careful monitoring is required to ensure no further self-harm occurs as patients may attempt to further complete their plan even while under active medical care.

DISPOSITION PLANNING

Not all patients with self-harm need hospitalization or immediate psychiatric evaluation. Initial evaluation should determine the need for medical admission for treatment of potential medical or surgical emergencies related to traumatic wounds or ingestions. If medical admission is not needed, attention should then focus on determining the presence or absence of suicidal intent associated with the patient's injury. Patients with ongoing suicidal ideation require psychiatric evaluation and hospitalization, though the majority of patients with NSSI can be cleared for discharge given the lack of suicidal intent inherent to the definition of this condition. Low-risk patients with minimal injuries, documentation of lack of suicidal intent, and access to outpatient resources may be safely discharged with a plan for close follow-up. This is a crucial step in the patient process as involuntary hospitalization may make the patient reluctant to seek health services for future injuries or in the setting of suicidal intent. Overall, establishing a safety plan is the best form of action to take in those with NSSI. This may be difficult in a time-sensitive setting but can put the patient on a positive clinical course. This includes addressing triggers/warning signs to self-harm, coping strategies (exercise, writing, music, etc.), resources for follow-up, and addressing positive support such as family and friends. It is also important to attempt to counsel removal of objects they use to self-harm, such as knives, lighters, ropes, etc.

In patients who are referred, primary treatment is in the form of dialectical behavior therapy, cognitive behavioral therapy, or psychotherapy. This is in addition to motivational interviewing to help patients find their underlying purpose for engaging in self-injurious behavior. Definitive intervention listed above is dependent on resources in the area and the level of those trained at local psychiatric facilities.

CASE RESOLUTION

After taking a detailed history from EMS, you sit down in the room with the patient. Setting aside your papers and pen, you take time to assure the patient that you are there to address both his medical and psychiatric needs. Your open approach leads the patient to disclose his recent social stressors, including increased demands at work and concerns about job security. He discloses a longstanding history of NSSI, including cutting and burning his extremities during adolescence as a way to manage his emotional pain. On direct questioning regarding his intention for his self-injurious behavior today, he confirms that he had no intention of harming himself and is not having any suicidal ideation currently.

His physical exam reveals a hemostatic wound on the left arm in addition to multiple old well-healed scars bilaterally. You irrigate the wound copiously with saline, suture it appropriately, and provide anticipatory guidance for wound care, suture removal, and expected healing. You order a tetanus vaccination given that he cannot recall his most recent vaccination date. The patient is calm and thankful for your help, though frustrated to be facing the return of old self-injury coping mechanisms. Given his lack of suicidal intent, you feel comfortable allowing him to return home with his roommate, who has come to the ED to support him. You make a specific plan for him to follow up at a local mental health clinic the following day for further psychiatric support.

KEY POINTS TO REMEMBER

- Self-harm or NSSI involves intentional damage to the body without suicidal intent.
- Medical evaluation and stabilization of the acute injury should be prioritized, followed closely by evaluation for psychiatric concerns.
- History should focus ascertaining the presence or absence of suicidal intent in order to establish a safe disposition for the patient.
- For the majority of patients with NSSI, referral for close outpatient follow-up with mental health resources is appropriate.

Further Reading

Hooley JM, Fox KR, Boccagno C. Nonsuicidal self-injury: Diagnostic challenges and current perspectives. *Neuropsychiatr Dis Treat*. 2020;16:101–112.

Kerr PL, Muehlenkamp JJ, Turner JM. Nonsuicidal self-injury: A review of current research for family medicine and primary care physicians. *J Am Board Fam Med*. 2010;23:240.

Lloyd-Richardson EE, Perrine N, Dierker L, Kelley ML. Characteristics and functions of non-suicidal self-injury in a community sample of adolescents. *Psychol Med*. 2007;37(8):1183–1192.

Walsh B. Clinical assessment of self-injury: A practical guide. *J Clin Psychol*. 2007;63:1057.

9 No License to Kill

Jay Brenner

R.R. is a 36-year-old man who presents to the ED complaining of homicidal ideation toward his girlfriend and mother. He says that he believes in the "two yoke" theory and that he has "four flaws." He is worried that one of his flaws would be killing the other "yoke," referring to his girlfriend. His physical exam reveals a disheveled appearance and a foul odor but is otherwise unremarkable, and his vital signs are normal. His mental status exam reveals that he has active homicidal ideations.

What do you do now?

THE HOMICIDAL PATIENT

Homicidal patients can stoke anxiety in the emergency physician (EP) charged with their care. On one hand, the disposition seems straightforward: Homicidal patients present a risk to others and therefore must be involuntarily admitted. On the other hand, the EP might worry that the patient is homicidal toward them or staff. While this is unlikely, an additional question of duty to warn the person toward whom they intend harm may also arise. Before offering specific guidance on these and other questions about the homicidal patient, we must first consider the underlying causes of the patient's homicidality, which may provide a source of our empathy for them.

Assessment

Historically, most homicidal patients have underlying psychosis. One study reviewing 110 patients who were involuntarily admitted for psychiatric treatment found that 16% were homicidal, and 89% of these patients were found to be psychotic.[1] A more recent study, however, suggested that patients reporting homicidal ideations are more likely to have depression than psychosis. It reviewed 251 patients who were involuntarily admitted for psychiatric treatment, 13 of whom (5.2%) were homicidal. Eleven of the 13 patients had a DSM-5 disorder, 9 had a depressive disorder, and 8 had a substance use disorder. Ten of the 13 were also suicidal. Eight of the 13 had active medical problems that required intervention in the ED. These included alcohol intoxication, hematuria, seizure, shoulder dislocation, abdominal pain, CHF exacerbation, and hyperglycemia.[2]

The assessment of a homicidal patient should include a prior history, collateral information, means, a plan, and medical screening. The psychiatry assessment can include the Historical, Clinical, and Risk Management-20 (HCR-20) (Table 9.1), which has been studied in psychiatry residents performing interviews on mock homicidal patients and validated as a predictor of recidivism.[3] This screening tool may provide a more standardized method for interviewing.

Duty to Warn

Many states have red-flag laws allowing physicians to notify law enforcement when patients are placed on an involuntary hold. R.R. would have

TABLE 9.1 **Historical, Clinical, and Risk Management-20 (HCR-20)**

Historical items	H1 Previous violence
	H2 Young age of first violent incident
	H3 Relationship instability
	H4 Employment problems
	H5 Substance use problems
	H6 Major mental illness
	H7 Psychopathy
	H8 Early maladjustment
	H9 Personality disorder
	H10 Prior supervision failure
Clinical items	C1 Lack of insight
	C2 Negative attitudes
	C3 Active symptoms of major mental illness
	C4 Impulsivity
	C5 Unresponsive to treatment
Risk management items	R1 Plans lack feasibility
	R2 Exposure to destabilizers
	R3 Lack of personal support
	R4 Noncompliance with remediation attempts
	R5 Stress

From: Wong L, Morgan A, Wilkie T, Barbaree H. Quality of resident violence risk assessments in psychiatric emergency settings. *Can J Psychiatry.* 2010;57(6):375–380.

met this criterion if he had had access to firearms. While not relevant to this adult patient, the American Academy of Pediatrics considers it best practice to screen for access to firearms in all adolescents, in part because 90% of homicides in adolescents aged 15 to 19 are firearm related.[4] *Tarasoff v. Regents of the University of California* set a precedent for the EP to notify law enforcement about homicidal intentions. If R.R. had mentioned a specific target of his homicidality by name and was discharged while still homicidal, breaching confidentiality would have been warranted.

Staff Safety

Management of the agitated patient is discussed elsewhere in this book, but it would be remiss not to address the increasing phenomenon of violence in the ED. One hundred percent of nurses have reported verbal assault and 82% physical assault over the course of their careers.[5] It is important that ED workers use de-escalation techniques at the first notice of agitation, such as higher-volume speech or hand gestures. Medications and restraints may become necessary. EPs should consider reporting any assault, even though the patient who incited it may have been psychotic. Sixty-five percent of healthcare workers who have experienced violence in the ED have not reported the incident.[6]

CASE RESOLUTION

In the case of R.R., he had no history, and collateral information was unavailable from either the girlfriend or the mother, toward whom he was feeling homicidal as well. He denied access to firearms, and he had made no mention of a plan other than to use his bare hands somehow. It was apparent that his thought content was disorganized, and his delusions were fixed and non-bizarre. His medical screening exam was unremarkable, as were his EKG and laboratory studies. An HCR-20 was performed; the EP noted a history of previous violence, relationship instability, major mental illness, lack of insight, impulsivity, lack of personal support, and stress. This tally of risk factors helped to improve the coordination of care with the inpatient mental health team. The EP discussed the case of R.R. with the psychiatry service on call, and they accepted him to the mental health unit on an involuntary status. He was discharged 5 days later, no longer feeling homicidal. (It should be noted that there is a more detailed Version 3 of the HCR-20 available for use as well.[7])

In conclusion, patients presenting to the ED with homicidal ideations frequently have psychosis, depression, or both. They should be screened for medical conditions as all patients with mental health complaints are, their risk should be assessed, and they should have an appropriate disposition. Additionally, special consideration should be given to the nature of their threats and whether further warnings to identified parties should be made.

> **KEY POINTS TO REMEMBER**
>
> · Most patients on an involuntary hold are not homicidal.
> · Most homicidal patients were historically psychotic, but most homicidal patients now are depressed.
> · Most homicidal patients are also suicidal.
> · Most homicidal patient have active medical problems.

References

1. Stern TA, Schwartz JH, Cremens MC, Mulley AG. The evaluation of homicidal patients by psychiatric residents in the emergency room: A pilot study. *Psychiatr Q.* 1991;62:333–344.
2. Maniaci M, Burton MC, Lachner C, et al. Patients threatening harm to others evaluated in the emergency department under the Florida Involuntary Hold Act (Baker Act). *South Med J.* 2019;112(9):463–468.
3. Wong L, Morgan A, Wilkie T, Barbaree H. Quality of resident violence risk assessments in psychiatric emergency settings. *Can J Psychiatry.* 2010;57(6):375–380.
4. Li CN, Sacks CA, McGregor KA, et al. Screening for access to firearms by pediatric trainees in high-risk patients. *Acad Pediatr.* 2019;19(6):659–664.
5. Tadros A, Kiefer C. Violence in the emergency department. *Psychiatr Clin North Am.* 2017;40(3):575–584.
6. Zun L. Care of psychiatric patients: The challenge to emergency physicians. *West J Emerg Med.* 2016;17(2):173–176.
7. Douglas KS, Hart SD, Webster CD, et al. Historical-Clinical-Risk Management-20, Version 3 (HCR-20v3): Development and overview. *Int J Forens Mental Health.* 2014;13:93–108.

10 Patient Is "Out of Control!"

Brian L. Springer

A 32-year-old male is brought in to the ED by
EMS with police assistance. His sister called
911 after noting that he was exhibiting bizarre
behaviors, wandering in the street and shouting
obscenities. She stated that he has a history
of cocaine abuse and schizophrenia and is not
compliant with his medications. On police and
EMS arrival, the patient was clearly agitated
and nonsensical and had begun to take off his
clothing out in the street. He seemed oblivious
to the presence of others and did not respond
to commands to sit on the ground. The medics
noted the patient was profusely diaphoretic.
Concerned about an acute medical emergency,
they asked the police to assist in restraining the
patient for an examination. As soon as contact
was made, however, he became combative and it
took multiple officers and medics to restrain him.
He continued to fight en route to the hospital. On
ED arrival he is agitated, screaming nonsensical
phrases, and diaphoretic and feels hot to the
touch. His blood glucose is 148. He is tachycardic
(HR 170) but BP could not be obtained due to his
combative status.

What do you do now?

EXCITED DELIRIUM SYNDROME

The clinical features of excited delirium syndrome (ExDS) were described in the 1800s and have been referred to by multiple other names, such as Bell's mania, exhaustive mania, lethal catatonia, and agitated delirium. In the 1970s it became associated with acute cocaine intoxication and psychosis, when ingested packets broke open in the bodies of smugglers. Seizures, coma, and death often followed. "Excited delirium" was first described in the modern literature in 1985 as the sudden onset of bizarre, paranoid, and violent behavior, associated with unexpected physical strength and hyperthermia. Fatal collapse occurred within minutes to hours of restraint. Again, most cases were linked to intoxication with stimulant drugs such as cocaine, methamphetamine, and phencyclidine (PCP). Psychiatric or systemic illness was sometimes felt to be a contributing factor. Many cases involved a struggle with law enforcement, including physical, chemical, or electrical control measures. Autopsy failed to yield a definitive cause of death. Currently, there are multiple definitions of excited delirium, none of which is universally recognized. It remains a clinically based syndrome, prone to much subjectivity in the scientific literature. It has been argued that excited delirium is not a valid diagnosis and that the term is used as a means of deflecting the investigation of in-custody deaths away from the actions of law enforcement personnel, with the goal of exonerating law enforcement and covering up police brutality. Excited delirium and ExDS are not recognized as exact diagnoses in the ICD-10. A patient may be diagnosed with cocaine delirium or delirium from a specific or unspecified stimulant or other psychoactive substance, but not with ExDS per se.

In 2009, the American College of Emergency Physicians published the *White Paper Report on Excited Delirium Syndrome.*[1] The purpose of the review study behind the white paper was threefold: to determine or disprove the existence of excited delirium as a disease; to determine the characteristics that help identify the presentation of excited delirium and the risk of death; and to look at current and emerging methods of control and treatment. The authors proposed a definition based on a syndromic approach wherein ExDS is identified by the presence of distinctive clinical and behavioral criteria recognizable in the premortem state. They noted that while potentially fatal, in some cases ExDS is amenable to early therapeutic interventions. The syndrome is characterized by delirium, agitation, and hyperadrenergic autonomic dysfunction, often in the setting of acute-on-chronic substance abuse or severe mental illness. The clinical features recommended by the authors are neither consistently seen in other studies nor mandatory for ExDS to be present; additionally, the criteria are not seen with the same frequency between studies and case series.[2]

PATHOPHYSIOLOGY

The common pathologic manifestation is delirium with multiple under-lying associations: psychiatric illness, psychiatric medication withdrawal, stimulant abuse, and metabolic disorders. What ultimately leads to ExDS is unknown and likely differs between cases.[3] Current literature hypothesizes that high levels of endogenous catecholamines related to exertion and stress, combined with concomitant stimulant abuse plus physical struggle or re-straint, result in hypoxia, hyperkalemia, acidosis, and autonomic dysfunc-tion. The abnormal response of the body leads to dysregulation dopamine homeostasis in the brain.

Dopamine mediates the perceived importance of environmental events and stimuli, and dopaminergic hyperactivity is linked to the symptoms of mania and psychosis. Cocaine blocks the dopamine transporter protein, prolonging dopamine receptor stimulation leading to behavioral activation. Chronic abuse of cocaine, methamphetamine, and other psychostimulants (such as ephedrine, MDMA, and bath salts) results in sensitization through increased dopamine transmission and prolonged receptor stimulation. Failure of dopamine regulation in cases of psychostimulant abuse, ex-treme mental stress, or an underlying psychiatric condition leads to agi-tation, delirium, and violent behavior. Neuroanatomic links between the brain and other organ systems result in distinctive cardiorespiratory and thermal dysregulation, allowing the development of hyperthermia and car-diac dysrhythmias.

The role of catecholamine surge resulting in hyperadrenergic state and acidosis is debated. A study comparing stress biomarkers in ExDS patients found significantly higher levels of cortisol in the ExDS arm compared to other agitated ED patients and a control arm of volunteers exercised to ex-haustion, physically restrained, and stressed by threats of application of a conducted energy weapon.[4] Studies looking at acidosis and catecholamine levels in simulated law enforcement encounters show that physical exertion tasks (sprinting, punching a heavy bag) generate greater changes than less lethal exposures such as oleoresin capsicum (OC) spray or Tom A. Swift Electric Rifle (TASER).[5,6] Therefore, physical resistance may put ExDS patients at greater risk than less lethal exposures. Acidosis leads to myocardial irritability and dysfunction, and catecholamine surges can cause lethal dysrhythmias. Unrecognized occult conduction abnormalities such as long QT syndrome may be unmasked, with resulting dysrhythmia and cardiovascular collapse. In addition, vasodilation associated with exertion results in decreased venous return when muscle activity ceases (i.e., the combative patient is restrained), reducing cardiac output and coronary artery perfusion at a time when elevated catecholamine levels increase heart rate and myocardial oxygen demand.

INCIDENCE

With no standardized definition of ExDS, determining its exact incidence is impossible. Prevalence varies widely based on the case definition and the context in which the episodes are described. Settings include EMS encounters, police encounters, ED or hospital patients, and forensic studies. Forensic literature looks at ExDS as a diagnosis of exclusion based on autopsy, with little discussion about survivors. ExDS is relatively uncommon among EMS encounters as a whole, with severe cases documented in less than 2 cases per 10,000 advanced life support calls.[2,3] Rates of ED presentation vary greatly, even among busy urban systems. The highest prevalence reported lies around 2.5% to 3% of patients transported by EMS.[3,7] Among agitated patients presenting to the ED, those who have symptoms of delirium have much higher rates of adverse events, including intubation, hypotension, and need for admission.

While police use of force is rare given the high incidence of citizen–police encounters, the presence of ExDS in cases that require use of force is disproportionately high. Depending on the criteria used, signs of ExDS are present in greater than 3% of use-of-force encounters, with as many as 15% (1 in 6) of individuals undergoing use of force having three or more clinical signs at that time.[2,8] Individuals with a greater number of clinical features of ExDS are less likely to have alcohol intoxication, more likely to have evidence of drug intoxication and emotional distress, and appear to be at higher mortality risk. The actual mortality rate for ExDS remains unknown. High estimates of 8% to over 16% are likely overestimated due to the absence of a clear definition and publication bias in the forensic literature.[2] The mortality rate is probably much lower, with one retrospective study showing a significant decline in restraint-related deaths attributed to ExDS over the past several decades. The authors speculate this reflects increased awareness of ExDS by police and EMS and decreased use of prone positioning for restraint, but they caution that the patient death rate in the study was so low overall as to limit any conclusions.[9]

Lacking a consensus definition, specific etiology, or single anatomic feature, ExDS is described by its epidemiology, common clinical presentation, and usual course. The presenting symptom cluster varies. It is the combination of delirium, psychomotor agitation, and physiologic excitation that differentiates ExDS from processes that result in delirium alone, or from individuals who are agitated and violent but not delirious.

In the prehospital setting, the features most often associated with ExDS are:

- Constant or near-constant physical activity with a lack of tiring
- Increased/abnormal pain tolerance
- "Superhuman" strength
- Tachypnea
- Diaphoresis
- Tactile hyperthermia
- Noncompliance/failure to respond to police presence

Other less common features include disrobing, nudity or inappropriate clothing, and an unusual attraction to glass, mirrors, or other reflective surfaces. Among a large Canadian cohort, subjects with three or more features were involved in 1 of 11 use-of-force encounters, and individuals with six or more features were involved in 1 in 66 use-of-force encounters.[10] The majority of patients in the cohort did not die, countering concerns that ExDS is a contrived condition to excuse improper procedure or excessive force following in-custody deaths. This also counters older literature on ExDS where death was part of the definition. As mentioned, this likely reflects publication bias looking specifically at fatal cases.[2]

Patients who die tend to die suddenly, often following physical, chemical, or electrical control measures, and with no clear anatomic cause of death noted on autopsy. Along with the clinical features mentioned above, fatal cases of ExDS include the following:

- Male gender
- Mean age mid-30s
- Destructive or bizarre behavior, including violence toward inanimate objects, that generate a call to police
- Suspected use of psychostimulants or history of psychostimulant abuse
- History of or suspected psychiatric illness
- Sudden cardiopulmonary collapse following a struggle and restraint, or shortly after a period of quiescence
- Inability to be resuscitated on scene

The differential diagnosis for ExDS covers a wide range of disease states associated with altered mental status. Prolonged observation combined with extensive testing may be required to uncover the underlying diagnosis. Several disease states deserve mention. Diabetic hypoglycemia may resemble intoxication and result in violent behaviors. Diagnosis can be made with bedside glucose testing. Classic and exertional heat stroke may result in tactile hyperthermia and delirium. A significantly elevated core temperature should prompt initiation of rapid cooling. Thyroid storm may result in hyperthermia and altered mental status, and thyroid function testing should be included in a comprehensive workup. Serotonin syndrome and neuroleptic malignant syndrome are associated with mental status changes, neuromuscular hyperactivity, and autonomic hyperactivity and may be difficult to differentiate from ExDS, as well as from each other.

RECOGNITION AND TREATMENT

Patients experiencing ExDS can go from combative to a perimortem state without warning. The key to effective treatment is early recognition. Without a gold-standard test, clinicians must use clinical judgment and act expediently if clinical indicators of the syndrome are present. While there is no strong evidence that sedation improves outcomes or prevents death, diminishing catecholamine surge and metabolic acidosis appears essential for positive short-term outcomes.

Prevent patients from injuring themselves or others. Have adequate staffing at the bedside, to include nurses, technicians, and security personnel. While physical restraint is often required, remember that in fatal cases cardiac arrest often follows a physical struggle. Be ready to quickly supplement physical restraint with appropriate medications. Supportive measures should target specific signs and symptoms. IV fluids can address fluid loss from elevated temperature, hyperventilation, and diaphoresis. Measured or tactile hyperthermia should be addressed through cool IV fluids and external cooling via ice packs or cooling blankets. If feasible, severe hyperthermia may be treated with cold-water immersion, especially if exertional heat stroke is part of the differential diagnosis.

Three classes of medication are of use when managing ExDS: benzodiazepines, antipsychotics, and dissociative agents. Benzodiazepines administered through the IV, IM, interosseous, or intranasal route have a rapid onset, working in minutes. They bind to GABA receptors and create an inhibitory response, which is ideal in patients with stimulant intoxication. The primary disadvantage is respiratory depression, which may be synergistic if alcohol or other sedative medications have been ingested. Antipsychotics can be used alone or in conjunction with benzodiazepines. First-generation antipsychotics such as haloperidol and droperidol are associated with QT prolongation, and droperidol was sidelined for years following a 2001 FDA black box warning. Recent studies have shown it to be safe and efficacious for treating agitated patients in the prehospital and ED settings. When doses greater than 2.5 mg are used, cardiac monitoring should be instituted once feasible. Ketamine is a dissociative anesthetic that prevents the higher brain centers from perceiving visual, auditory, or painful stimuli. When administered IM, onset of action is about 5 minutes, making it ideal for gaining control of agitated patients. Side effects include hypersalivation, nausea, emergence reactions, and rarely laryngospasm. Obviously, these patients may be critically ill and are at risk for rapid deterioration, warranting hospitalization and ongoing observation and treatment, initially in the intensive care setting.

CASE RESOLUTION

With police assistance, you and your staff place the patient in 4-point restraints and quickly administer haloperidol and lorazepam IM. The patient calms down enough to establish an IV, obtain labs and administer fluids. His temperature is 99, so you forgo rapid cooling measures. He is maintaining his airway and shows sinus tachycardia on the monitor. After an additional dose of haloperidol and lorazepam, the patient is calm enough to obtain an EKG which is nonspecific. His labs show mild rhabdomyolysis without renal failure. He is admitted for further observation, with a plan for psychiatric consultation.

KEY POINTS TO REMEMBER

- ExDS is a clinical diagnosis without a gold-standard test.
- Early recognition is critical. Delirium combined with psychomotor agitation and autonomic dysfunction should raise suspicion for ExDS.
- Early, aggressive supportive care, including rapid institution of anxiolytic pharmacotherapy, is associated with improved outcomes and reduced mortality.

References

1. American College of Emergency Physicians (ACEP) Excited Delirium Task Force. White paper report on excited delirium syndrome. 2009. https://www.acep.org/administration/ems-resources/

2. Gonin P, Beysard N, Yersin B, Carron PN. Excited delirium: A systematic review. *Acad Emerg Med.* 2018;25(5):552–565.

3. Vilke GM, DeBard ML, Chan TC, et al. Excited delirium syndrome (ExDS): Defining based on a review of the literature. *J Emerg Med.* 2012;43(5):897–905.

4. Vilke GM, Mash DC, Pardo M, et al. EXCITATION study: Unexplained in-custody deaths: Evaluating biomarkers of stress and agitation. *J Forens Legal Med.* 2019;66:100–106.

5. Ho JD, Dawes DM, Nelson RS, et al. Acidosis and catecholamine evaluation following simulated law enforcement "use of force" encounters. *Acad Emerg Med.* 2010;17(7):e60–e68.

6. Ho JD, Dawes DM, Nystrom PC, et al. Markers of acidosis and stress in a sprint versus a conducted electrical weapon. *Forens Sci Int.* 2013;233(1–3):84–89.

7. Miner JR, Klein LR, Cole JB, et al. The characteristics and prevalence of agitation in an urban county emergency department. *Ann Emerg Med.* 2018;72(4):361–370.

8. Hall CA, Kader AS, McHale AMD, et al. Frequency of signs of excited delirium syndrome in subjects undergoing police use of force: Descriptive evaluation of a prospective, consecutive cohort. *J Forens Legal Med.* 2013;20(2):102–107.

9. Michaud A. Restraint-related deaths and excited delirium syndrome in Ontario (2004–2011). *J Forens Legal Med.* 2016;41:30–35.

10. Baldwin S, Hall C, Bennell C, et al. Distinguishing features of excited delirium syndrome in non-fatal use of force encounters. *J Forens Legal Med.* 2016;41:21–27.

Further Reading

Gonin P, Beysard N, Yersin B, Carron PN. Excited delirium: A systematic review. *Acad Emerg Med.* 2018;25(5):552–565.

Riddell J, Tran A, Bengiamin R, et al. Ketamine as a first-line treatment for severely agitated emergency department patients. *Am J Emerg Med.* 2017;35(7):1000–1004.

Vilke GM, Bozeman WP, Dawes DM, et al. Excited delirium syndrome (ExDS): Treatment options and considerations. *J Forens Legal Med.* 2012;19(3):117–121.

Vilke GM, DeBard ML, Chan TC, et al. Excited delirium syndrome (ExDS): Defining based on a review of the literature. *J Emerg Med.* 2012;43(5):897–905.

11 Two for the Price of One

Dana Sacco

A 30-year-old male presents to the ED with suicidality. He says that he has been feeling down lately and that life isn't worth living. He endorses regular alcohol consumption. When asked if he has a plan, the patient says he has been thinking about overdosing on medications. You notice that the patient smells of alcohol. Vital signs are within normal limits. Physical exam shows mild slurring of speech and unsteady gait consistent with intoxication, and a depressed affect; the exam is otherwise unrevealing. You are caring for a patient who has expressed suicidal ideation and who also appears to be intoxicated. You wonder if the patient is feeling suicidal only because he's drunk and if he will still endorse suicidal ideation when he sobers up. You do not know if he has a history of alcohol dependence.

What do you do now?

CO-OCCURRING MENTAL HEALTH AND SUBSTANCE USE DISORDER DIAGNOSES

Many patients with substance use disorders (SUDs) also suffer from mental health diagnoses, and vice versa. The co-occurrence of both in a patient is referred to as *dual diagnosis*. About 40% to 60% of people with alcohol use disorder experience depression, and among individuals with major depression approximately 16.5% have an alcohol use disorder and 18% have a drug use disorder.[1]

The presentation of affective symptoms (e.g., sadness, irritability, lack of energy, sleeplessness, mania) in a patient with a primary mood disorder versus in a patient whose mood disorder is secondary to substances (i.e., substance induced) will appear to be very similar. However, the patient with the substance-induced mood disorder will display symptoms that are temporally related to ingestion or withdrawal from the substance.

This case describes a patient with acute alcohol intoxication who presents with suicidality; however, this could have been a presentation of depression, mania, or psychosis with acute intoxication of methamphetamine, opioids, cocaine, or any other illicit substance. In all of these cases, substances complicate the management of a patient with a psychiatric complaint.

Which Came First, the Chicken or the Egg?

When treating a patient in the ED, it can often be difficult to disentangle whether a patient with an SUD has subsequently developed mental health symptoms (e.g., depression, mania, psychosis) or whether a patient with a primary mental health disorder has subsequently turned to substances. As emergency medicine providers, we see a patient at one snapshot in time. A patient's prior history (if present in the medical record) may be enlightening but often will not be available. However, from the perspective of the ED provider, it may not be necessary or possible to fully tease this apart, but it will be necessary to acknowledge that a patient is suffering from both.

Treating the Whole Patient

Managing patients with both a mental health diagnosis and an SUD diagnosis requires a multidisciplinary approach and is more likely to be successful when a patient's family or other social support structure is also involved. The ideal outpatient scenario may involve the patient's primary care physician, an addiction specialist, a therapist, and an outpatient substance abuse clinic. The role of an SUD clinic varies depending on the substance involved, and for opioids it may also include medication-assisted therapy (MAT) in the form of buprenorphine or suboxone (buprenorphine plus naloxone). In the case of other SUDs (e.g., alcohol), ongoing counseling and peer-group support may be useful as well.

Involving social work in the ED can help to connect a patient to these resources. ED social workers are likely to have knowledge of SUD clinics and detox centers and in some cases can help a patient to make these appointments.

Mental Health Complaints in the Setting of Acute Intoxication

If a patient's suicidal ideations (or symptoms of mania, depression, or psychosis) resolve upon sobering up, it is likely that the patient will not need inpatient psychiatric care. However, these patients continue to be vulnerable, especially in the setting of ongoing substance abuse, and it is critically important to provide outpatient resources for treatment of their SUD.

Challenges in Treating Patients with Mental Health Complaints and Concomitant SUD

The use of substances is likely to make it difficult for a patient to keep appointments, take medications, and follow the treatment plan reliably. For this reason, a multidisciplinary team should be involved in a patient's care and, when possible, a patient's social network should be enlisted for support as well.

ED providers are often dismissive of a patient's acute mental health complaints when the patient is also observed to be under the influence of substances. However, patients with concomitant diagnoses are also at increased risk of suicide.

CASE RESOLUTION

Because the patient expressed suicidal ideation, he was placed on clinical watch and allowed to metabolize the alcohol back to sobriety. Once sober, he could engage in a reasonable conversation about his problem with alcohol and expressed that he wanted help and did not actually want to end his life. Social work provided the patient with appropriate substance abuse and mental health resources.

When possible, it is important to understand the patient's past psychiatric and mental health history. Both psychiatry and social work should be involved as needed, and it is vitally important to obtain their help with connecting the patient to resources following discharge from the ED. This patient population poses unique challenges, and a multidisciplinary approach to care is the most likely to be successful.

KEY POINTS TO REMEMBER

- Patients with suicidality in the setting of substance abuse require clinical observation for safety, the same as if there were no substances involved.
- Involve an addiction specialist, which is likely to be done on an outpatient basis. Social work should be able to provide resources.
- When necessary, refer patients to substance disorder clinics that will take patients without insurance and possibly also without a telephone.
- Use physical restraints in the ED only as a last resort.

Reference

1. Revadigar N, Gupta V. Substance induced mood disorders. StatPearls. 2021. https://pubmed.ncbi.nlm.nih.gov/32310347/

Further Reading

Goldsmith RJ, Garlapati V. Behavioral interventions for dual-diagnosis patients. *Psychiatr Clin North Am.* 2004;27(4):709–725. doi:10.1016/j.psc.2004.07.002

Quello SB, Brady KT, Sonne SC. Mood disorders and substance use disorder: A complex comorbidity. *Sci Pract Perspect.* 2005;3(1):13–21. doi:10.1151/spp053113

Revadigar N, Gupta V. Substance induced mood disorders. StatPearls. 2021. https://pubmed.ncbi.nlm.nih.gov/32310347/

Tolliver BK, Anton RF. Assessment and treatment of mood disorders in the context of substance abuse. *Dialogues Clin Neurosci.* 2015;17(2):181–190. doi:10.31887/DCNS.2015.17.2/btolliver

12 "My Neighbors Are Harassing Me"

Ryan E. Lawrence

A 22-year-old male arrives via ambulance, accompanied by police for "making threatening statements." He called the police from home complaining that he was in danger, that neighbors were harassing him, and that he would "take care of it myself" unless the police intervened. The patient is unkempt, with poor eye contact and flat affect. He responds to questions by shrugging his shoulders and asking, "When can I leave?" His parents arrive and are visibly concerned. They report he was previously a gregarious university student. Over the past year he stopped attending classes and stopped socializing. He unenrolled from school and moved back home with his parents. They explain, "At first we thought he just needed a break and some time to set new goals." At home he became increasingly withdrawn, spending most days in his room smoking cannabis and looking out the window. The parents add, "He began complaining about the neighbors 6 months ago. We asked him to see a doctor, but he refused."

What do you do now?

SCHIZOPHRENIA

This patient exhibits several features suggestive of schizophrenia, including a nonspecific prodrome, a decline in function, negative symptoms (social withdrawal, reduction in grooming, flat affect, and poor eye contact), and positive symptoms (paranoia about the neighbors), with a duration lasting more than 6 months. Some alternative psychiatric diagnoses that should be considered include substance-induced psychotic disorder; major depression with psychotic features; bipolar disorder, current episode depressed, with psychotic features; and delusional disorder. Some medical conditions that can cause psychotic symptoms include infection, autoimmune disease (e.g., lupus cerebritis), endocrine disorders (e.g., hypothyroidism), and neurologic disorders (e.g., epilepsy, multiple sclerosis).

All patients presenting with new psychotic symptoms should receive a medical workup to assess for reversible causes. This evaluation usually includes a medical and psychiatric history (including assessment of travel, hobbies, work history, and family history), a physical exam, a CBC, a metabolic panel, LFTs, thyroid function tests, vitamin B12 levels, testing for syphilis and HIV, and drug screening. Lumbar puncture is not routinely performed.

Brain imaging at this stage is controversial. Neuroimaging studies are a major component of schizophrenia research. CT and MRI studies have revealed abnormalities involving brain structures and white matter connections. Functional neuroimaging studies have suggested altered metabolic or hemodynamic activity in several brain regions. PET, SPECT, and MR spectroscopy studies have provided a window into the role of brain neurotransmitters and receptors in schizophrenia. However, the clinical role of neuroimaging in the workup of presumed schizophrenia is currently limited to excluding other causes of psychosis. Neuroimaging should be performed if there is high suspicion for a neurologic condition (e.g., seizures, a preexisting neurologic disorder, known brain pathology, a family history of neurologic disorder), a history of head trauma, acute onset of symptoms, or evidence of delirium.

A safety assessment is critically important for this patient, especially since he was brought in by police for making vaguely threatening statements. A safety assessment should include clarification of any statements he made

("When you said you would take care of it yourself, what did you have in mind?"). It should also assess for other known risk factors for violence or self-harm, such as prior behaviors that involved harm to self or others, prior or current thoughts of harming self or others, access to weapons (especially access to guns), and active substance use. Obtaining collateral history from the parents (or other close associates) adds to the quality of the safety assessment. While there is no formula for quantifying the patient's risk level, and nobody can be expected to predict the future, understanding (and documenting) the risk factors and protective factors is necessary for meeting the standard of care and can be quite useful when formulating a treatment plan. Whether or not the patient meets criteria for inpatient hospitalization will vary according to regional definitions and regulations articulating what constitutes dangerousness to self, dangerousness to others, or inability to function.

Treatment

The initial treatment plan should be informed by several principles. First and foremost is the goal of engaging the patient in treatment. Facilitating a treatment alliance, implementing shared decision-making, and placing the individual's goals at the center of the treatment plan can all serve to keep the person engaged in treatment and focused on recovery. Patient experiences of coercion, feeling that treatment plans are not consistent with personal goals, or feeling that treaters are not listening to concerns sufficiently can all compete with this goal of engagement.

When arranging outpatient follow-up, providers should note that programs specializing in first-episode psychosis have been especially successful at improving outcomes. These programs often include multidisciplinary teams with low caseloads, an ability to meet with clients in a variety of settings, manualized cognitive behavioral therapy, individualized crisis-management plans, family counseling, and psychoeducation. Increasingly these programs also use peer supports to promote engagement and decrease stigma, as well as computer-based technologies (e.g., online chat platforms) to increase opportunities for clinical contact and support.

An antipsychotic medication (D2 dopamine antagonist) is very likely to improve this patient's positive symptoms (paranoia about the neighbors). Starting a medication sooner rather than later is important because a longer duration of untreated psychosis is associated with a worse prognosis. Guidelines indicate the most important consideration when selecting a medication is the side-effect profile. For this reason, olanzapine is specifically not recommended in first-episode psychosis, due to very high rates of weight gain, hyperlipidemia, and diabetes. For this patient, aripiprazole 5 mg daily could be a reasonable selection, since the metabolic and motor side-effect burden is relatively low, and it is available as a generic, which increases affordability. Many other antipsychotics could also be appropriate; all should be started at a low dose. Antipsychotic effect will likely take approximately 1 week to appear. Within 2 weeks, the patient and treater should have a reasonable understanding of how effective the medication will be for the patient. In most cases the patient will be encouraged to stay on the medication for at least a month before trying alternatives. When symptom remission is achieved, guidelines suggest remaining on the medication (at the lowest effective dose) for at least a year and possibly longer.

The initial treatment plan should address the patient's cannabis use. An association exists between cannabis use and the development of schizophrenia, especially among persons who use cannabis during adolescence and who consume greater quantities. Reducing or stopping cannabis altogether may help reduce the psychotic symptoms. At the very least, stopping cannabis will simplify the differential diagnosis and reduce confounding factors, if the psychosis proves difficult to treat. A brief intervention in the ED setting might include psychoeducation, an assessment of the individual's readiness to change, and linkage to substance use treatment programs if the individual is receptive.

Discussing the diagnosis and treatment recommendations with the patient and family can be extremely challenging, even for experienced providers. It can be very difficult to judge when and how to have the conversation, and there is genuine controversy surrounding how much to disclose at this stage. There are reasons to consider having a frank conversation about the diagnosis: Treatment recommendations will make more sense to the patient, the patient and family members can begin educating themselves about the illness and the supports available, and the patient may discover the diagnosis anyway if it is written on clinical paperwork or if antipsychotic medication is prescribed. At the same time there are reasons to exercise caution: A diagnosis of schizophrenia carries considerable stigma and is often surrounded by misinformation, individuals might lack insight or be unreceptive to the conversation, there is no definitive confirmatory test, and this is a one-time evaluation, which leaves some room for alternative diagnoses such as substance-induced psychotic disorder.

One approach to the conversation might include the following elements:

- Offer reassurance: "I have seen situations like this before and I have some ideas that could help."
- Assess receptivity: "Are you interested in having a conversation about how I am putting the pieces together?"
- Identify the key data points using the patient's (or the family's) vocabulary: "Your parents told me you withdrew from school, you are socializing far less than you used to, you have been very worried that the neighbors are harassing you, and I can see you are not shaving or brushing your hair."
- Introduce a diagnosis and offer some basic teaching (many specialists would use the language of psychosis rather than schizophrenia at this stage): "These symptoms make me think you are experiencing psychosis. This is a medical condition that leaves your brain vulnerable to misinterpreting signals and events. In your case it is causing you to feel very unsafe."
- Offer hope and link to care: "There are some very good treatments available. Most people benefit from a combination of medication and talk therapy. I would like to connect you with a clinic where there are people who would love to partner with you, to help you get back to your life, and to reach your goals."

CASE RESOLUTION

A safety assessment revealed no acute safety concerns. The patient accepted a first dose of aripiprazole 5 mg in the ED with no adverse effects and received a 2-week prescription. An outpatient psychiatry clinic provided an appointment for later that week. The parents agreed to bring him back to the ED if any safety concerns reappeared. He was discharged home.

- The most important goals for the encounter are to assess for safety and to attempt to engage the patient in treatment.
- Placing the patient's goals at the center of the treatment plan will increase the likelihood of keeping the patient engaged in treatment.
- Routine medical workup for a presumed onset of schizophrenia should focus on excluding reversible causes of psychosis.
- Antipsychotic medication selection following a first episode of psychosis is based primarily on the side-effect profiles of the available drugs. Avoid olanzapine because of metabolic side effects.
- Clinical programs specializing in treating a first episode of psychosis have produced better outcomes than treatment as usual.

Further Reading

Alvarez-Jiménez M, Parker AG, Hetrick SE, et al. Preventing the second episode: A systematic review and meta-analysis of psychosocial and pharmacological trials in first-episode psychosis. *Schizophr Bull.* 2011;37(3):619–630.

Dixon LB, Holoshitz Y, Nossel I. Treatment engagement of individuals experiencing mental illness: Review and update. *World Psychiatry.* 2016;15:13–20.

Farooq S, Green DJ, Singh SP. Sharing information about diagnosis and outcome of first-episode psychosis in patients presenting to early intervention services. *Early Interv Psychiatry.* 2019;13(3):657–666.

Keating D, McWilliams S, Schneider I, et al. Pharmacological guidelines for schizophrenia: A systematic review and comparison of recommendations for the first episode. *BMJ Open.* 2017;7:e013881.

Keshavan MS, Collins G, Guimond S, et al. Neuroimaging in schizophrenia. *Neuroimag Clin North Am.* 2020;30(1):73–83.

Ortiz-Medina MB, Perea M, Torales J, et al. Cannabis consumption and psychosis or schizophrenia development. *Int J Soc Psychiatry.* 2018;64(7):690–704.

13 The Fatigued IT Worker

Gary Khammahavong and Mitchell Kosanovich

A 32-year-old woman presents to the ED with low energy and feeling down. She reports increased fatigue. She was laid off from her job at an IT firm 2 months ago and has been having a hard time getting back on her feet. She states that today she felt particularly down as it was the anniversary of her mother's death. She had thoughts about harming herself over the past few days but did not have any plans. She has a previous history of self-harm where she has cut her wrists. She had been an avid painter, but now she does not find the same joy in it as she had before. She reports previous marijuana and cocaine use and drinks a glass of wine a night. She denies hallucinations. She has no significant past medical history. Her father was bipolar and her mother had hypothyroidism. On examination, the patient is normotensive with HR of 80. Other than healed scars on her wrists, the physical exam is within normal limits.

What do you do now?

DEPRESSION

While the diagnosis for this patient is depression, the differential can be quite broad. She has a significant previous history of recreational drug use. She also drinks daily. Her family history is also noteworthy for both a psychiatric disorder and an organic cause of dysthymia. Another area that complicates the case is her previous history of self-harm, as well as her suicidal ideation. A thorough questioning and examination of the patient's suicidal ideations as well as her risks of suicide are warranted given her history, as this will dictate her disposition.

The differential for a patient who comes in with fatigue is broad and can include psychiatric disorders as well as organic, medical disorders. Initial assessment should be based on clinical exam. Does the patient appear to be intoxicated? Is the patient coherent or does the patient appear confused? If so, it will require waiting until he/she is not altered or is clinically sober again to reassess his/her suicidal ideation or depressive state. In addition to the clinical exam, a thorough history should be taken from the patient regarding his/her medical and social history. Certain medical conditions, such as hypothyroidism or Parkinson's disease, can cause some depressive symptoms. Medications, such as steroids or interferons, can also induce them.

A quick screening test that can be used for patients in whom you suspect depression is the Patient Health Questionnaire (PHQ)-2. The PHQ-2 is an abbreviated version of the PHQ-9, which has been used in the primary care setting as a screening tool for depression, but is much shorter and easier to administer. Answers can be provided in a yes-or-no fashion, and a positive answer can be an indicator for clinical depression. The test itself is quite specific, with a sensitivity of 76%.[1] Other screening tests and clinical tools that can be used are the Ask-Suicide-Screening Questions (ASQ), Manchester Self Harm Rule (MSHR), and Risk of Suicide Questionnaire (RSQ), which all have good sensitivities as screening tools for depressive and suicidal ideations.[2-4] These tests and clinical tools are helpful as they can be quickly administered and evaluated with only a handful of questions.

Another helpful way of evaluating patients is through the mnemonic **SIGECAPS**, which stands for *S*leep, *I*nterest, *G*uilt, *E*nergy, *C*oncentration, *A*ppetite, *P*sychomotor function, and *S*uicide. Changes in these symptoms, such as decreased sleep or interest, increased sleeping, change in appetite, or confusion, can be signs that a person is going through depression. If a patient has five or more of these symptoms daily for at least 2 weeks, it is possible the patient may be having a depressive episode. Using the PHQ-2, PHQ-9, or other mentioned screening tools, along with these symptoms, can be a good way to screen and assess the severity of a patient's possible depression.

Regarding the workup for this patient, bloodwork and testing may be necessary. Per the American College of Emergency Medicine, obtaining lab work is not necessary unless the physical exam and history warrant it. However, in the acute ED setting, lab tests may aid in evaluating for organic as well as toxicological causes. The findings will also be helpful for the psychiatry team. Lab tests that can be beneficial as screening tests are noted in Table 13.1. These tests help to evaluate for possible organic causes of the patient's depressed mood or fatigue. Other tests to consider are CT head, especially in elderly patients, or lumbar puncture if there is concern for a meningeal infection. If the patient is on antiepileptic medications or already on psychiatric medications such as lithium, it may be also be beneficial to check the levels of these medications. The benefits of the EKG, as well as checking drug levels, are to help assess if there are toxic causes of the patient's symptoms. Patients who are intoxicated on alcohol or other drugs can display symptoms consistent with depressed mood or suicidality. Patients who are withdrawing from certain drugs or coming down from a high, such as cocaine, can also appear to be clinically depressed. In these cases, a patient's symptoms can be attributed primarily to his/her drug intoxication or withdrawal and will need to be reassessed again when clinically sober.

For a patient who comes to the ED for depressed mood and fatigue, the above workup can help move you toward a final disposition for the patient. If a psychiatry team is available for evaluation of the patient after the workup has been completed, it may be beneficial for them to evaluate him/her. If a psychiatry team is not available, then the final disposition will be dependent on how great of a risk the patient poses to himself/herself or others. This is where the assessment of the patient's suicide risk is paramount. This involves questioning the patient regarding his/her suicidal ideation. Is there a previous history of suicide attempts? Does the patient

TABLE 13.1 **Labs and Testing for Screening of Depression Patients in the ED**

Test	Rationale
Complete blood count	Assess infection, anemia
Basic metabolic panel	Assess electrolyte abnormalities, glucose levels
Liver function panel	Assess possible liver damage, dysfunction if concerned for cirrhosis or acetaminophen overdose
Pregnancy test	Rule out pregnancy-associated mood disturbances
TSH/free T4	Assess thyroid function for clinical hyper- or hypothyroidism
Urine drug screen	Assess if possible drug ingestion or withdrawal as cause of symptoms
Alcohol level	Assess if patient has alcohol intoxication causing mood disturbance
Urinalysis	Assess for infection
Acetaminophen level	Assess for ingestion of acetaminophen if concern for overdose and altered mood
Salicylate level	Assess for ingestion of salicylates if concern for overdose and altered mood
EKG	Can be used as screening tool if there is concern for overdose

have a plan? If so, what is the plan? If the patient is at risk of harming himself/herself, the patient will meet criteria for psychiatric admission if the patient is agreeable to admission. Depending on where you practice, if you feel strongly that the patient is at risk of harming himself/herself, you may be able to involuntarily admit the patient to a psychiatric facility. If the patient is not at immediate risk for suicide, the patient may be discharged with close follow-up. The patient should be provided with good resources for community outreach and psychiatric programs.

For pediatric patients, the assessment of depression and suicidality should be done in a similar fashion to performing an assessment in an adult.

Roughly 77% of patients between the ages of 0 and 19 years will have some type of healthcare visit or contact a year before they commit suicide.[5] The assessment of a pediatric patient should be done without the parent or guardian in the room; other than this, the assessment is the same for an adult. A thorough history and physical should be performed and lab work that is deemed necessary should be obtained as well.

Patients with depression will typically need to be started on an antidepressant such as a selective serotonin reuptake inhibitor (SSRI). Generally, these medications should not be started in the ED as it is difficult to follow up with these patients. Other treatment options include tricyclic antidepressants (TCAs) and cognitive behavioral therapy.

CASE RESOLUTION

Given this patient's previous history of self-harm as well as her suicidal ideation, she demonstrates signs of possible depression based on your screening tests. She appears to be clinically sober and does not have any active suicidal ideation. Based upon your examination and discussion with her, you defer testing. You do speak with her again and she states that she has a boyfriend in whom she confides regularly. She states that she feels safe at home. She is amenable to following up with a psychiatrist. You find out through your resources that there is an outpatient crisis center that is open 24 hours a day, as well as a hotline. You provide her with this information, as well as the follow-up information for a psychiatrist. As she is clinically stable, not intoxicated, does not have any active suicidal ideation, and is not at risk to herself or others, you feel she is safe for discharge. She is discharged in stable condition from the ED.

KEY POINTS TO REMEMBER

· Rule out organic causes. Many medical conditions can cause fatigue as well as other vague symptoms such as feeling down. Even if the patient clinically appears to be depressed, organic causes need to be ruled out.
· Assess for drug levels and intoxication. Drug and alcohol intoxication as well as hyper-therapeutic drug levels can cause depressed mood or suicidal ideation.

- Patients who are altered or intoxicated should be reassessed when not altered or when clinically sober.
- Determine the patient's suicide risk and whether he/she has a plan. If there is a plan and there is an immediate risk for suicide, this is a reason for psychiatric admission.
- Depending on your clinical practice setting, the patient may be admitted involuntarily if you are strongly concerned for his/her immediate risk of suicide and the patient is unwilling to be admitted.
- In pediatric patients, a similar workup should be performed, as well as a thorough evaluation of stressors, socioeconomic circumstances, and risk factors.
- Attempt to assess pediatric patients without their parent(s) or guardian in the room.

Further Reading

ACEP Emergency Medicine Practice Committee. Care of the psychiatric patient in the emergency department: A review of the literature. 2014. https://www.acep.org/globalassets/uploads/uploaded-files/acep/clinical-and-practice-management/resources/mental-health-and-substance-abuse/psychiatric-patient-care-in-the-ed-2014.pdf

Betz ME, Caterino JM. Suicide. In: Walls R, Hockberger R, Gausche-Hill M, eds. *Rosen's Emergency Medicine: Concepts and Clinical Practice*. 9th ed. Philadelphia: Elsevier; 2018:1366–1373.

Hoyer DA, David E. Screening for depression in emergency department patients. *J Emerg Med*. 2008;43(5):786–789.

Maurer DM. Screening for depression. *Am Fam Physician*. 2012;85(2):139–144.

Patten SB, Barbui C. Drug-induced depression: A systematic review to inform clinical practice. *Psychother Psychosom*. 2004;73(4):207–215.

Zun LS, Nordstrom K. Mood disorders. In: Walls R, Hockberger R, Gausche-Hill M, eds. *Rosen's Emergency Medicine: Concepts and Clinical Practice*. 9th ed. Philadelphia: Elsevier; 2018:1346–1352.

14 An Energetic College Student

Lauren J. Curato

A 20-year-old female is brought to the ED by police from the local university. She was found alone in the school's quad at 1 a.m., inappropriately dressed and lecturing about current events. She announces she is the daughter of a prominent politician and intends to sue you and the school, then transitions to the subject of climate change. She is pacing the room, does not participate in your attempts to obtain a medical history, and is easily distracted by efforts to change her into a gown. She is fully oriented. She is afebrile with HR 92 and regular. The remainder of the physical exam is normal. Further history obtained from her roommate reveals the patient has not slept in over 3 days but still went to the gym for hours each day, cleaned their dorm room, and went on several dates. The patient has no past medical history other than one episode of depression in high school; she is not on medications. There is no history of drug or alcohol abuse.

What do you do now?

BIPOLAR DISORDER

This is a previously healthy college student presenting with a significant behavioral change from baseline that is now impairing her ability to function appropriately in society. Her symptoms include psychomotor agitation, tangential speech, grandiose thinking, distractibility, and increased levels of energy, all concerning for a manic episode with psychotic symptoms. Her prior history of depression makes this likely to be a case of bipolar I disorder with a current manic episode.

The differential diagnosis of psychosis is broad and consists of medical, substance-induced, and psychiatric causes. Medical disorders including head trauma, thyrotoxicosis, systemic lupus erythematosus, seizures, and infection as well as medication-induced psychosis (e.g., steroids) need to be considered. Substance-induced psychosis can be caused by stimulants (amphetamines, cocaine, synthetic cathinones) and psychedelics. Even withdrawal from agents such as alcohol or other sedatives can cause psychosis. Psychiatric causes include depression with psychotic symptoms, anxiety disorders, schizophrenia, and bipolar disorder.

When evaluating a patient with psychosis or depression it is important not to miss a reversible cause of the behavioral change. This necessitates a thorough medical, psychiatric, and social history that is aided by collateral information from friends and family. A physical exam that evaluates for trauma, infection, toxidromes, and focal neurologic deficits is crucial.

Emergency physicians are frequently asked to perform routine laboratory tests and neuroimaging prior to the psychiatric evaluation. It is recommended that testing be guided by prior medical and psychiatric history and examination. Patients with new-onset psychosis are a subset of patients who may benefit from testing to help rule out other potential causes of psychosis. One study has found that psychosis due to an underlying medical condition accounted for more than half (54.7%) of the patients presenting to their ED with a first episode of psychotic symptoms.[1] Lab testing could include CBC, BMP, TSH, rapid plasma reagin, and serum alcohol levels. The undifferentiated psychotic patient may also benefit from neuroimaging such as CT brain. This is especially important if there are focal neurologic findings on exam to rule out intracranial hemorrhage and mass lesion. If no focal neurologic deficit is present, an individual assessment of risk factors can guide brain imaging.

Patients who present to the ED with acute psychosis are frequently agitated, which may be exacerbated by the typical chaotic surroundings of the department. The American Association for Emergency Psychiatry has published a consensus statement for de-escalating the agitated patient. It stresses the importance of creating a safe environment for the patient (and staff) and broaching the topic of medication administration early in the visit, so the patient can remain calm and participate in his/her care. Suggesting or offering anxiolytic medication can give patients a sense of control that they likely otherwise feel they have lost. Physical restraint should be considered only as a last resort.

Bipolar disorder is a lifelong illness involving episodes of mania or hypomania and major depression. Mania is the hallmark of bipolar I disorder, while hypomania defines bipolar II. Bipolar I is the current description of the classic "manic-depressive" illness. The difference between the two forms is the severity of the mania. According to the DSM-5, in bipolar I, the mood disturbance is sufficiently severe to cause marked impairment in social or occupational functioning or to necessitate hospitalization to prevent harm to self or others, or there are psychotic features. As emergency providers, we typically see bipolar patients when they have acute mania or severe depression with or without suicidal ideations. Hypomanic (bipolar II) patients rarely seek care in the ED unless there is concern for worsening of their condition. The diagnostic criteria for depression in bipolar disorders are the same as those of major depressive disorder, which will be discussed in Chapter 13.

Typically, the manic patient is brought to the ED by family, law enforcement, or EMS. It is important to obtain collateral information from these individuals; information such as onset of symptoms, recent behavior, possible triggers, drug use, knowledge of previously prescribed medications, and past medical and family history of psychiatric disorders is key. The circumstances that led the patient to be brought in to the ED can be varied. While some may appear psychotic during a manic episode, others may present with suicidal ideation. Suicidality can occur during any phase of bipolar disorder, but patients are at higher risk of suicide during a severe depressive episode. It is thought that the lifetime risk of suicide is at least 15 times greater in bipolar patients than in the general population. When patients are manic, they do not perceive themselves to be unwell and frequently refuse treatment. They will have an elevated mood and can seem like the life of the party one moment but quickly transition toward belligerence and irritability the next. Frequently they are more talkative than usual and their speech is pressured, so much so that the clinician cannot interpret what they are saying. During this time, they have an inflated sense of self-esteem (grandiosity) and can be distractible. Many manic patients have heightened energy and do not require sleep. It is important to note this is different from insomnia, when a person wants to sleep and cannot; in mania, patients have an actual decreased need for sleep. Some may get involved in a grand project such as writing a book (increased goal-directed activity) while others may engage in risky behaviors, for example unsafe driving, shopping sprees, poor investment choices, theft, drug or alcohol use, and sexual indiscretion (activities that have potential for painful consequences). It is not uncommon for acutely manic individuals to present to the ED as trauma patients. The common symptoms of mania can be summarized by the classic mnemonic DIG FAST, which is summarized in Figure 14.1.

In the ED, patients can present with decompensation of their bipolar disorder at any age, but the average age of onset of the disorder is 18 years. In the United States the lifetime prevalence is thought to be about 1% of the population, affecting both men and women equally. Bipolar disorder is known to be a very heritable disease. Studies have shown that the risk of bipolar disorder in a child or sibling of someone with the disorder is about 10%, and monozygotic twin concordance is approximately 40%.[2] Substance abuse is a known complicating factor both for the diagnosis and

---

DIG FAST

Distractibility   Flight of ideas
Irritability   Activity increased
Grandiosity   Sleeplessness
   Thoughtlessness

FIGURE 14.1 Mnemonic for the symptoms of mania

the treatment of bipolar disorder. Comorbid substance abuse is found in over 50% of patients with bipolar I. A diagnosis of bipolar disorder can only be made when the symptoms are present in the absence of substance use.

One special population to consider is the postpartum woman. Women with known bipolar disorder are at risk for decompensation during this period, and undiagnosed women at risk for bipolar disorder may show their first symptoms during the postpartum period.

In patients presenting with symptoms of new-onset mania or depression, ED clinicians may develop a working diagnosis, but ultimately the psychiatry team will make the diagnosis and determine long-term treatment. Our role is to optimize safety, break the cycle of the patient's behavior, and start to stabilize the patient's mood so he/she may participate in his/her care. Patients presenting with acute mania will require a much different approach than the calm, nonpsychotic patient who may be depressed and suicidal. Patients should be placed in a safe location, searched for any harmful objects, and changed into gowns that distinguish them as high risk from the general patient population. Some patients may require a staff member to sit with them and monitor them closely (one on one) to prevent self-harm. Others, who are calm and cooperative and not posing an imminent threat to themselves or others, can be grouped with patients who are also undergoing psychiatric evaluation. They can be monitored from a distance by security simply to prevent them from leaving the department.

Mania should be considered an acute medical emergency because if left untreated, patients may engage in behaviors that are harmful to themselves and others. Three categories of medications—neuroleptics, benzodiazepines, and mood stabilizers—are all commonly used in this phase of bipolar disorder.

Neuroleptic (antipsychotic) drugs are known to be effective in acutely manic patients and have the advantage of being available in parenteral form for agitated patients unwilling to take a pill. The typical antipsychotics, also known as first-generation antipsychotics (with the classic example being haloperidol), are very effective but do have the potential to cause side effects, including extrapyramidal symptoms such as dystonia and akathisia and tardive dyskinesia as well as QT prolongation and hypotension. Due to these side effects, they are not well tolerated for long-term treatment but can be beneficial in the acutely manic patient, in whom both the antipsychotic and sedating properties are wanted. The sedating property of the drug can help the patient sleep; this is important in manic patients who have not slept because the lack of sleep is believed to propagate the mania. The newer atypical, or second-generation, antipsychotics such as risperidone, olanzapine, ziprasidone, aripiprazole, and quetiapine are also very beneficial and tend to cause fewer dystonic side effects. Many of these medications are available in PO, oral disintegrating, and IM forms (both short acting and extended release). For patients not already taking long-term treatment for bipolar disorder, this class of medications seems to show effect for short-term resolution of symptoms.

Benzodiazepines have no anti-manic effect but can be used in combination to assist with sedation in the acutely psychotic patient and to reduce tension and improve sleep. Using haloperidol and a short-acting benzodiazepine such as midazolam or lorazepam IM is common practice in the agitated, psychotic patient in the ED. Olanzapine is noted to have the side effect of orthostatic hypotension, and there have been reports of cardiopulmonary depression when used in combination with benzodiazepines. It should be common practice to place any patient requiring immediate sedation with combined benzodiazepines and antipsychotic agents on cardiorespiratory monitoring.

Lithium and the anticonvulsants valproic acid and carbamazepine are oral mood stabilizers used in the treatment of bipolar disorder. All three have been shown to be effective but have slow onset and require patient compliance with PO therapy. Thus, treatment is usually initiated with an antipsychotic agent with the mood stabilizer added in as patient compliance permits. Initiation and selection of a new mood stabilizer should be left to psychiatric expert consultation. Patients presenting to the ED with acute mania will require inpatient psychiatric hospitalization to ensure safety, achieve mood stabilization, and institute an appropriate treatment plan. From the emergency physician's perspective, this patient represents an unsafe discharge, and the ultimate disposition will be admission.

The treatment of bipolar depression has been a dilemma in the psychiatry arena for years. Antidepressants used to treat unipolar depression have been thought to precipitate mania in bipolar patients. If an antidepressant is to be used, it is recommended that patients also take a mood stabilizer or antipsychotic agent. Initiation of treatment of bipolar depression in the ED should be done only with the assistance of psychiatric consultation.

The long-term natural course of bipolar illness varies with each patient. Many patients can go on to fully recover between episodes and maintain employment and functionality, while others have significant disability. As emergency physicians, it is important to remember our role in their long-term treatment: to ensure their safety, to ensure there is not an acute medical illness causing their symptoms, and to be their advocate when they cannot be their own.

CASE RESOLUTION

This patient had a past history of depression but has not been on medication. She has no other medical problems, she has no drug abuse history, and she was not believed to be acutely intoxicated. Her physical exam was not consistent with acute trauma nor any specific toxidrome, and there were no focal neurologic findings. The patient underwent lab tests, all of which were unremarkable for acute pathology. Brain imaging was deferred. Upon her initial evaluation, she was pacing the exam room but was cooperative. She was offered medication to help manage her restlessness, to which she was agreeable, and after 2 mg of PO lorazepam she was able to sleep. A psychiatry consultation was placed, at which point it was discovered that her deceased mother had a history of bipolar disorder. The patient was admitted to the psychiatric unit and started on olanzapine and lithium therapy. She was ultimately discharged and able to return to her college courses.

KEY POINTS TO REMEMBER

- Bipolar disorder is a lifelong illness that involves episodes of mania or hypomania and major depression.
- Symptoms of mania can be identified by recalling the mnemonic DIG FAST.
- Patients who are acutely manic, severely depressed, or suicidal are unable to care for themselves. They pose a threat to their

own safety and cannot be discharged from the ED. Psychiatric
consultation should be obtained and a plan for admission made.
Antipsychotics and mood stabilizers are the mainstays of
therapy in bipolar disorder.

References

1. Etlouba Y, Laher A, Motara F, et al. First presentation with psychotic symptoms to the emergency department. *J Emerg Med*. 2018;55(1):78–86.
2. Craddock N, Jones I. Genetics of bipolar disorder. *J Med Genet*. 1999;36:585–594.

Further Reading

Barnhill JW. *DSM-5 Clinical Cases*. Arlington, VA: American Psychiatric Association; 2014.

Klein LR, Driver BE, Miner JR, et al. Intramuscular midazolam, olanzapine, ziprasidone, or haloperidol for treating acute agitation in the emergency department. *Ann Emerg Med*. 2018;72(4):375–385.

Nazarian DJ, Broder JS, Thiessen MEW, et al. Clinical policy: Critical issues in the diagnosis and management of the adult psychiatric patient in the emergency department. *Ann Emerg Med*. 2017I;69(4):480–498.

Richmond JS, Berlin JS, Fishkind AB, et al. Verbal de-escalation of the agitated patient: Consensus Statement of the American Association for Emergency Psychiatry Project BETA De-escalation Workgroup. *West J Emerg Med*. 2012;13(1):17–25.

15 A Different Type of ABCs

Emily Donner and Brent Rau

A 43-year-old male presents to the ED with a complaint of abdominal pain. The patient has an extensive history of hospitalizations regarding similar complaints. On exam, you notice multiple healed linear scars on the patient's forearms. The patient demands abdominal imaging, even though he has been scanned 10 times over the past 4 months with no abnormality identified. You give him a one-time dose of fentanyl for pain. The patient then states, "You are the best doctor in the world. It is so nice that someone actually cares about me and knows what they're doing." After you find no acute pathology, you tell the patient he will not be getting any further opioid medication, and that he is stable for discharge to home. The patient's mood changes dramatically. He demands to be seen by another doctor and that you leave the room immediately. He is asking to get the hospital administration involved because he is tired of feeling abandoned and believes he needs admission for pain.

What do you do now?

PERSONALITY DISORDERS

This patient is exhibiting classic traits of borderline personality disorder. These patients have a strong need to feel connected with others. The best way to approach these patients is to validate their feelings and engage in conversation. This can place a great demand on your time, in a setting in which multiple patients compete for your attention. These patients often present with mild symptoms and demand more time, disrupting workflow.

Of particular importance, these individuals are at an increased risk for suicide, even when they are not currently endorsing any suicidal ideation. If possible, an attempt should be made to make sure the patient is not alone or in an isolated room. Once the patient is stabilized medically, the psychiatry staff should ideally be involved. These patients are often resistant to psychiatric evaluation, making these scenarios even more difficult.

Personality disorders are classified as Clusters A, B, and C. Although there may be many different types, a common thread runs through them all. A personality disorder is defined by the DSM-5 as a personality trait that impedes the ability to be flexible, causing maladaptation throughout social and occupational situations, thus hindering the ability to function in society. In patients suffering from this affliction, the relationship between the emergency doctor and the patient can be even more strained than it is when they see their primary care provider, with whom they've had a relationship for years. As the emergency physician, you are charged with developing a trusting relationship, communicating effectively, and treating appropriately in minutes to hours. A colleague of mine once told me, "If you dislike a patient within the first 10 seconds of meeting them, they probably have a personality disorder." Keeping this pearl in mind, informally pre-briefing (if you've been forewarned of the difficult patient in Bay 22) and debriefing, exhaling deeply, and checking in with yourself before and after the clinical encounter makes treating medical disorders in people with personality disorders much less stressful. The following is a brief summary of the classifications.

Cluster A: The Weird

Paranoid: A global theme of distrust. May accuse partners of infidelity without reason. Won't engage in office water-cooler chat because he believes Bill from accounting will use the information against him.

Schizoid: Detached. Family life? Sex? No thanks. Indifferent toward praise or criticism; chooses solitary activities above all else.

Schizotypal: This disorder encompasses a wide range of pathology, from magical thinking to paranoia. These individuals can even experience bodily illusions, so when a patient exclaims, "Your aura is a beautiful shade of purple! I can tell you're a good doctor," take the compliment and keep in the back of your mind you're likely treating someone with schizotypal personality disorder.

Cluster B: The Drama

Antisocial: A pattern of guiltless behavior and lack of remorse. Presents as conduct disorder as an adolescent (symptoms prior to 15 years of age). Psychopathy is at the extreme end of this spectrum. It might be what you're familiar seeing on a televised true crime documentary.

Borderline: Instability and impulsivity. Borderline personality disorder (BPD) is the most studied personality disorder and the one you are most likely to encounter during your clinical practice. Characterized by splitting: labeling others as "all good or all bad." Quick to interpret neutral comments or actions as negative, making objective medical care exceedingly difficult.

Histrionic: The classic example is walking into a patient room, to be greeted by sexual advances, while the patient is wearing lingerie or something of that nature. Individuals suffering from this personality disorder use physical appearance to draw attention to themselves and will often interpret relationships as more serious or intimate than they are.

Narcissistic: Strong need for attention and admiration. Hypothesized to correlate to patient–caretaker relationship, often caused by parental coldness or rejection. Often seen in high achievers, from physicians to politicians.

Cluster C: The Afraid

Avoidant: Will avoid activities for fear of criticism and ridicule. However, they DO desire personal relationships. An overall feeling of inadequacy.

Dependent: Lacks self-confidence to the point of engaging in activities the individual may deem unpleasant just to gain the approval of others. Will quickly attempt to start a new relationship when another ends—preoccupied by the total fear of being alone.

Obsessive-compulsive: Often hyper-focused on minor details. Classically a perfectionist and compulsory note taker who struggles with task switching. The behaviors of a patient with an obsessive-compulsive personality disorder align with personal values (ego-syntonic). This stands in contrast to obsessive-compulsive disorder, which is distressing to the patient (ego-dystonic). Although counterintuitive, patients can be prone to hoarding behavior, despite an obsession with control of their environment.

APPROACH TO TREATMENT

Most treatment approaches to personality disorders are based upon long-term goals, requiring multiple therapy sessions with a mental health professional whom the patient has learned to trust. It is best to have an open and frank discussion about the diagnosis with the patient, if you feel that a known psychiatric diagnosis is contributing to the presentation. With that being said, it would be improper to make a psychiatric diagnosis, particularly one involving personality disorders, in the ED, no matter how strong the inclination. Furthermore, keep in mind that patients are often cognizant of their idiosyncrasies, and the clinical relationship may change significantly if they detect your suspicion of a psychiatric contribution to their presentation. Screening tools, formal and informal, exist for personality disorders and may have clinical utility.

Questions should be posed in a sensitive and nonjudgmental manner. Treatment strategies vary depending on the disorder. With the goal of representativeness, we have chosen to focus on strategies to best manage patients presenting with BPD, as it is one of the disorders we encounter most frequently and is also the most studied. These individuals use EDs regularly, and we encounter these patients when they are in crisis and when they present for routine medical care.

Following is an informal screen for Cluster B personality disorder. Any positive answers increase the likelihood of its diagnosis:

- Do you lose your temper easily?
- Do you find you act on impulse often?
- Does your mood go up and down frequently?
- Do you like to be in the center of situations?

When patients present with acute agitation, all efforts should be made to calm them. Little evidence supports the use of any one pharmacologic agent; however, benzodiazepines are frequently used. Of course, these carry the significant risks of respiratory depression and hypotension. Typical antipsychotics are also a popular choice, although you may then be faced with treating subsequent dystonic reactions or akathisia. Recent studies have suggested the use of atypical antipsychotics as a first-line agent. In particular, a one-time dose of IM olanzapine has been increasingly effective, with only 16% of patients requiring a second dose.

New pharmacologic interventions for patients in BPD crisis are being studied. In addition to atypical antipsychotics, other interesting avenues being explored are highlighted here. Clonidine has been shown to ease inner tension as well as desires to commit behavior that may be self-injurious. A randomized controlled trial (RCT) has shown oxytocin administration reduces aggression and the perception of societal threats.[1]

Arguably, BPD patients who are presenting *not* in crisis are much more difficult to treat. The negative attitude of healthcare staff toward those with BPD has been demonstrated in multiple studies. The beliefs that these patients may be manipulative, lack proper communication skills, and are often time-consuming cases to manage are largely thought to be the root of such feelings. The lack of compassion and feeling of negativity toward these patients only exacerbates their potential volatility, which in turn may lead to an increase in use of aggressive measures that otherwise may have been avoided. Unnecessary use of physical restraints and overuse of sedating medications increase rates of patient harm and, ultimately, liability.

To avoid these aforementioned outcomes, training programs should be implemented to educate hospital staff on the nature of this condition. Doing so has proven to increase compassion and patience in the medical community. Workshops should be provided for all individuals involved in the patient's healthcare timeline. This includes pre-hospital workers, as patients in crisis often arrive to the ED by EMS. Social workers are reputed to show the most positive attitude toward these patients. Early involvement of social work and a multidisciplinary approach is paramount.

Although treating these patients in crisis may represent the clear majority of BPD patients we encounter, a focus on providing patients with proper outpatient follow-up is key. Connecting them with sources for psychotherapy has been proven to decrease impulsivity, aggressiveness, and suicidal attempts/self-injury and, ultimately, ED visits. The type of therapy associated with the most positive outcomes is dialectical behavior therapy (DBT). This is a form of cognitive behavioral therapy (CBT) that focuses on emotions, to develop healthy means to cope with stress and forming relationships.

CASE RESOLUTION

You reassure the patient that you have his best interests in mind. You take a seat, make sure to lean forward, and maintain eye contact, reminding yourself that physical communication can be as important as verbal communication in showing empathy. You say, "I cannot imagine what you are going through. You seem to really be in pain. Can you please tell me your primary concern today? What exactly was the incident or moment you decided you had to go to the emergency room?" The patient becomes tearful. He admits that he had been under a significant amount of stress at home. He recently broke up with his long-term girlfriend and was laid off from his job. He goes on to say he had been feeling worthless and was hoping pain medication would help to numb his emotions and bring him some sort of relief. You thank the patient for his honesty.

Social work is asked to participate in the patient's care, providing him with resources for psychiatric centers, counselors, and numbers he can call if he is in crisis. He is appreciative that someone had truly heard him. He firmly denies any suicidal ideation or access to firearms at home. He has no thoughts of harming others. Ultimately, he is able to be discharged home with his new resources.

Not all patient scenarios like this will resolve in such an idyllic manner. The reality will often leave you exhausted, frustrated, and questioning how you could have approached cases such as this differently. Despite this, doing your best to approach these patients with an open mind, with the priority of making them feel heard and validated, is rewarding and can make the difference for patients who are willing and open to making a change.

There is much research to be done in terms of management and effective approaches to patients with personality disorders, especially in the emergency setting. With so many of the disorders left unstudied, we have large gaps in our breadth of knowledge, leaving many individuals with suboptimal care. The focus should be on educating the medical community on the nature of these diseases to encourage compassion and patience. Affirming the patient's complaints and feelings is paramount in effective communication and problem solving.

The pharmacologic options for psychiatric crisis most commonly used are benzodiazepines and typical antipsychotics, with a push toward atypical antipsychotics like olanzapine. If possible, before discharge, patients should receive referral to a psychiatric professional for further evaluation, ideally one who specializes in treating personality disorders.

KEY POINTS TO REMEMBER

- Validate the patient's feelings.
- Show compassion and patience.
- Encourage education in psychiatric conditions among hospital staff.
- Try your best to establish appropriate follow-up prior to discharge; it will save you an ED visit later!

Reference

1. Bertsch K, Gamer M, Schmidt B, et al. Oxytocin and reduction of social threat hypersensitivity in women with borderline personality disorder [published

correction appears in Am J Psychiatry. 2013 Oct 1;70(10):1218]. *Am J Psychiatry.* 2013;170(10):1169–1177. doi:10.1176/appi.ajp.2013.13020263

Further Reading

American Psychiatric Association. Diagnostic and Statistical Manual of Mental Disorders. *5th ed. Arlington, VA: American Psychiatric Association; 2013.*

Bertsch K, Gamer M, Schmidt B, et al. Oxytocin and reduction of social threat hypersensitivity in women with borderline personality disorder [published correction appears in Am J Psychiatry. 2013 Oct 1;70(10):1218]. *Am J Psychiatry.* 2013;170(10):1169–1177.

Chapman AL. Dialectical behavior therapy: Current indications and unique elements. *Psychiatry.* 2006;3(9):62–68.

Mirza I, Rahman A. Psychiatric emergencies in personality disorders. In: Thara R, Vijayakumar L, eds. *Emergencies in Psychiatry in Low- and Middle-Income Countries.* Delhi, India: Byword Books; 2011:155–164.

Shaikh U, Qamar I, Jafry F, et al. Patients with borderline personality disorder in emergency departments. *Front Psychiatry.* 2017;8:136. doi:10.3389/fpsyt.2017.00136

16 The Deadly D's of the Elderly

Jennifer Cullison

An 81-year-old female is brought in to the ED by EMS after a friend went to her house and found her confused at home. The patient is sitting on the edge of the ED bed, looking perplexed, with a small abrasion to her forehead and incontinent of urine. She is fidgeting, staring around the room, looking in her bag, and picking at the blood pressure cuff and bed sheet. When asked questions she becomes more agitated, uncooperative, and does not follow many commands. On your evaluation the patient admits that she hasn't felt well in 3 days but wants to go home and have a glass of wine. She can only recall her name and date of birth. She tells you she is sure she is lost and needs to find her mother. While the nurse attempts to obtain vitals the patient becomes combative. The patient has past medical history of osteoporosis, recurrent UTIs, and depression. She takes amlodipine, citalopram, and acetaminophen. She has no known allergies. The patient lives independently, drinks three glasses of wine per day, and usually manages own daily life activities. Vitals are HR 86, BP 150/70, RR 14, SpO_2 95% on room air, temp 37.3°C.

What do you do now?

MENTAL ILLNESS IN THE ELDERLY

A chief complaint of confusion or altered mental status must trigger an evaluation in a systematic manner beginning with vital signs. Patients with abnormal behavior typically have bedside testing for hypoglycemia and hypoxia. Sepsis can present with thermoregulation symptoms such as fever or hypothermia. Hypertensive encephalopathy is a diagnosis of exclusion but cannot be forgotten. If alcohol or drugs are of concern, do not forget Wernicke's encephalopathy and all other ingestion toxidromes.

Acute neurologic disorders, such as meningitis and subarachnoid hemorrhage, can also present with confusion. Ischemic, basilar ischemic, and bilateral thalamic stroke could also present with altered mental status. Seizures may present with a transient postictal state or an ongoing subclinical decreased mentation. The most frequent disorders causing altered behavior are common systemic illness such as UTIs, pneumonia, and medication adverse effects. Virtually every medical condition is capable of causing confusion that could appear as delirium, including electrolyte disorders, endocrine diseases, thyroid disease, myocardial infarction, and CNS masses.

Delirium and confusional states are among the most common mental disorders encountered in patients with medical illness, especially among the elderly. In general, delirium can be found wherever there are sick patients.

A primary dilemma the clinician faces is differentiating delirium from depression or dementia. History and clinical course are important in differentiating these syndromes. This is especially difficult with many patients who present in the ED from long-term care facilities or nursing homes. Even when there are known cognitive deficits, it must be determined if the current medical condition is caused instead by delirium. Inattention is usually not a feature of mild to moderate dementia, and its presence supports delirium. Depression, mania, and nonorganic psychotic disorders typically do not arise in the settings of medical illness. Further, altered level of consciousness is typically not present in dementia or depression. At times, the diagnosis can be quite difficult when patients are uncooperative and symptoms are subtle, but because of the life-threatening nature of delirium, one should err on the side of treating the patient as delirious until further information is gathered.

The causes of delirium are broad and can include medical conditions, substance intoxication, withdrawal or medication side effects, or an alteration that cannot be explained by an established neurocognitive disorder. Delirium as a geriatric syndrome is inherently multifactorial and develops as a result of interactions between predisposing risk factors and noxious insults.

Psychiatric disorders such as depression, bipolar disorder, and schizophrenia represent another group of diagnoses in which patients may present with altered mentation. The clinical features of older bipolar patients differ from those of younger patients, and the number of geriatric bipolar patients is expected to increase as the average life expectancy increases over the next several decades.[1] The minimum age to define geriatric bipolar disorder is generally 60, and this includes both aging patients whose mood disorders presented earlier in life and for the first time later in life. Geriatric bipolar patients are predominately female as compared to the younger generation, which has a 1:1 predominance. It is also theorized that the causes of late-onset geriatric bipolar disorder may differ from those of a younger generation, shown by observations of CNS pathology occurring in more late-onset bipolar patients. Some examples supporting the disease process of geriatric bipolar disorder include reduced volume of gray matter structures, white matter hyperintensities, and biochemical changes.[2] Geriatric bipolar disorder may be also attributed to the progressive CNS deterioration of aging, evidenced by signs of inflammation, oxidative stress, and mitochondrial dysfunction.[3]

DESCRIPTIONS OF PSYCHIATRIC ILLNESSES IN THE GERIATRIC POPULATION

Delirium is an acute disorder of attention and cognitive function that can arise at any point in the course of an illness. It is characterized by alteration of consciousness and cognition with reduced ability to focus, sustain, or shift attention. It develops over a short period and may fluctuate during the day. It is often the only sign of a serious underlying medical condition, especially in older persons who are frail or have underlying dementia.

The prevalence of delirium on admission can range from 10% to 40%. Delirium is the most common postoperative complication among older adults, with rates of 15% to 52%.[4] Higher rates are seen in the ICUs, and 80% of terminally ill patients become delirious before death. The diagnosis is often missed, more so in the hypoactive type because of poor clinical manifestation.

Bipolar disorder in both geriatric and younger patients is characterized by episodes of major depression, mania, and hypomania. It is associated with cognitive deficits affecting attention, abilities to switch tasks, memory, and verbal fluency. This is in comparison to the clinical presentation of delirium, which can vary but usually presents with psychomotor behavioral insults such as hyperactivity or hypoactivity. Increased sympathetic activity and impairment in sleep duration have been described as hyperactive, hypoactive, and mixed. The hypoactive form is often unrecognized but is more common with older hospitalized patients; it is associated with a poorer overall prognosis.

Geriatric bipolar disorder can be associated with dementia, and the risk of dementia in these patients is more than twice as high as those without preexisting bipolar disorder. A concern in bipolar geriatric patients is the higher rate of suicide. A study of 220 mixed-age adult bipolar patients followed for 34 to 38 years found that the rate of completed suicide was 12 times higher in patients than in the general population, and this risk remained constant over the lifespan up to age 70.[5]

EVALUATION OF PSYCHIATRIC EMERGENCIES IN THE ELDERLY

The initial clinical evaluation must begin with a psychiatric history and mental status exam. Clinicians must assess depressive, manic, and hypomanic symptoms in their review of systems.

Delirium can be a life-threatening emergency. Initial evaluation is largely based on establishing the patient's baseline cognitive functioning. A detailed history from a reliable informant, such as a spouse, caregiver, or child, may need to be obtained. The clinician should seek to clarify the acuity of mental status change and inquire about any clues to the underlying cause. The cardinal historical features of delirium are acute onset and fluctuating course, in which symptoms tend to come and go over a 24-hour period.

Delirious patients in the ED may pose a challenge if they become agitated. Patients may fall or pull out IV lines, catheters, and endotracheal tubes. Any patient who is not alert and oriented, has behavior changes while in the ED, or appears altered should be formally assessed for delirium.

The Society for Academic Emergency Medicine Task Force has recommended delirium screening as a key quality indicator for emergency geriatric care. Tools such as the Brief Confusion Assessment Method (bCAM) and Confusion Assessment Method (CAM) are both useful in the ED. Cognitive changes are assessed through clinical observation and special testing. Categories of inattention, disorganized thinking, altered level of consciousness, psychomotor agitation, hallucinations, and sleep–wake cycles are all integral components and are best measured by the CAM. The CAM was created in 1990 and designed to allow non-psychiatric clinicians to diagnose delirium quickly and accurately following brief formal cognitive testing.[4] This tool also served as the foundation for the bCAM developed for ED patients.[6] Another useful ED test is the Short Blessed Test (SBT),[7] also called the Orientation-Memory-Concentration test. This weighted six-item instrument was originally designed to identify dementia. Conversely, no direct screening tool has been developed for geriatric bipolar disorder.

CAUSES OF PSYCHIATRIC EMERGENCIES IN THE ELDERLY

Delirium in elderly patients is rarely caused by a single insult but is typically due to interactions of multiple contributing factors. There are "predisposing factors," which make the individual more vulnerable, and there are "precipitating factors," which are the insults that cause the actual mental disturbances. In the ED, it is important to identify these, as the risk of delirium increases with each factor present.

Uncontrolled pain is commonly identified as a single delirium trigger. Unfortunately, emergency physicians are less successful at treating pain in geriatric patients, likely due to opioid prescribing concerns of sedation and delirium. Nonpharmacologic therapies to manage pain, including ice, elevation, and immobilization, should be considered.

Urinary retention can precipitate or exacerbate delirium, a disorder referred to as cystocerebral syndrome. Bladder distention may contribute to delirium via increased sympathetic tone and catecholamine surge triggered by tension on the bladder wall.[3]

Dehydration precipitates delirium in that it leads to cerebral hypoperfusion. Severe dehydration can also be a sign of severe neglect. Recognition of dehydration in elderly patients can be more challenging, as the physical findings of weight loss, decreased skin turgor, dry mucous membranes, tachycardia, and hypotension are unreliable in the geriatric population.

Environmental factors, even those on the small scale of the ED itself, may cause sensory overload, creating disorientation and worsening delirium. Frequent checks to ensure patients have not become tethered to devices and lines or tangled in bed sheets or blankets are important. Soiled briefs/garments may pose risks for worsening infections and create stress.

Polypharmacy is common in older adults and in many situations contributes to delirium. The Beers criteria (or Beers list) alerts clinicians about the dangerous side effects of medications. The Beers list, from the American Geriatrics Society, catalogs medications to be avoided in older adults. It emphasizes deprescribing unnecessary medications and helps to reduce polypharmacy. The medications commonly linked with delirium are those with anticholinergic properties. The effects of polypharmacy can be magnified during acute illness, with hepatic and renal dysfunction unexpectedly increasing half-lives and therefore increasing the effects of the medications.

MANAGEMENT AND TREATMENT OF GERIATRIC PSYCHIATRIC EMERGENCIES

Approaches to the treatment are threefold: (1) identify and treat the underlying cause, (2) eradicate or minimize contributing factors of delirium, and (3) manage the symptoms of current condition. A complete review of medication and supplement history should be performed, and the agents should be assessed for interactions. Laboratory assessments should be performed and diagnostic imaging reviewed. Treatment begins with nonpharmacologic approaches in all patients. These therapies can include reorientation, fluid repletion, feeding assistance, sensory correction, and pain management. Pharmacologic interventions should be reserved for emergencies in individuals whose behavior interferes with medically necessary care or poses a safety threat to the patient. Physicians must remember that all medications used to treat acute agitation and delirium can also worsen confusion, so they should always use the lowest doses and the shortest timeframes. No medication is currently approved by the FDA for the management of delirium, so the use of antipsychotics is off label. Medications such as antipsychotics and benzodiazepines are commonly used when the risks and benefits are weighed in patients with severe agitation. Benzodiazepines have a fast onset, and this can be critical for a patient who is exhibiting self-harm for whom no alternatives are available. Low-dose haloperidol has limited evidence to support its use for severe agitation and psychotic symptoms but may be used as needed in extreme situations. For the treatment of mania and hypomania in a bipolar geriatric patient, pharmacotherapy is generally used and there are first-line and second-line agents.

CASE RESOLUTION

Management of this case involved referral to psychiatry, a phone call to the primary physician, and a call to social work with concerns of safety at home and the ability to perform daily life activities. This patient's history included medical comorbidities of hypertension and depression, while living alone with symptoms of a UTI. The patient also consumed alcohol daily and took an antidepressant. Her tox screen was negative. The patient's PCP provides you contact information for the patient's daughter, whom you reach by phone. She speaks to her mother, and, with gentle persuasion, you are able to convince the patient to stay. She is admitted to the medical service.

KEY POINTS TO REMEMBER

- Delirium, dementia, and depression exist on a continuum; this blurs the diagnostic distinction, especially in geriatric patients.
- Three approaches to treatment are (1) identify and treat the underlying cause, (2) eradicate or minimize contributing factors of delirium, and (3) manage the symptoms of the current condition.

- Cast a wide net when evaluating elderly patients with altered mental status, as many of these patients have life-threatening illnesses.
- Caution should be advised when treating well-known patients in the ED, as complacency breeds contempt.

Further Reading

Carpenter CR, Bassett ER, Fischer GM, et al. Four sensitive screening tools to detect cognitive dysfunction in geriatric emergency department patients: Brief Alzheimer's Screen, Short Blessed Test, Ottawa 3DY, and the Caregiver-Completed AD8. *Acad Emerg Med.* 2011;18(4):374–384.

Leslie A, Wei, BA, Fearing MA, et al. The Confusion Assessment Method (CAM): A systematic review of current usage. *J Am Soc Geriatr.* 2008;56(5):823–830.

Sajatovic M, Chen P. Geriatric bipolar disorder: Epidemiology, clinical features, assessment, and diagnosis. UptoDate, 2020.

Sajatovic M, Chen P. Geriatric bipolar disorder: Treatment of mania and major depression. UptoDate, 2020.

Shenvi C. Assessing and man. 2015. https://www.aliem.com/delirium-in-older-adults/.

Singhai K, Suthar N, Gehlawat P. The 3 Ds of geriatric psychiatry: A case report. *J Family Med Prim Care.* 2020;9(5):2509–2510.

Thakrar A, Snell T, Prabhakar D. Delirious mania in a geriatric patient. *Prim Care Companion.* 2018;20(1):17102141.

17 Spiraling Out of Control

Purva Grover

A 9-year-old boy was in a quiet room at a local psychiatric day treatment program when he began threatening suicide and banging his head against the observation window. This caused his forehead to bleed. When staff attempted first aid, he attacked them, scratching one of them in the face and bending another's finger to the point of causing a deformity. He was then placed into four-point leather restraints and transported to your ED, where he is now growling and spitting at you and the ED staff. He is tachycardic and tachypneic, and BP could not be obtained because the patient is thrashing about. Your staff is apprehensive, and the parents at the bedside are extremely anxious.

What do you do now?

PEDIATRIC PSYCHIATRIC EMERGENCIES

The Center for Medicare and Medicaid Services specifies that restraints should be used only when patients become so aggressive or violent that their behavior is an immediate danger to their own safety on that of others. At this time, however, you can consider the following:

1. First and foremost, try to de-escalate the situation by attempting to calm the patient. Understandably, he is upset and is now in restraints and surrounded by strangers, and the situation is likely going to escalate quickly if he feels further threatened or helpless.
2. The parents at the bedside could be an invaluable resource in helping to calm the patient down. Sometimes, however, the presence of parents or loved ones can be a trigger to the patient. Read the room carefully.
3. Identify the right resources. Sometimes you will find that members of the ED staff are exceptionally good with bonding and reaching out to this patient population. If you have such people on your staff, bring them to this room.
4. If verbal de-escalation is not helping, and the patient is continuing to be agitated and seems at risk for hurting himself or hurting staff around him, then you will have to consider chemical restraint.

One of the best choices for reducing agitation in this otherwise un-complicated patient is a low-dose sedative available in PO form, such as midazolam. Diphenhydramine and other mild sedatives can be effective for mild agitation, but midazolam is usually more effective for moderate agitation, particularly when there is a concern for escalating behavior. However, if delirium is suspected, benzodiazepines should be avoided be-cause they can disinhibit the child and worsen the delirium. Olanzapine and ziprasidone are atypical antipsychotics that are available in PO and IM forms and are useful for agitated patients with symptoms of delirium or psychosis. Haloperidol is a typical antipsychotic also available in PO and IM forms and is useful for agitation with delirium or psychosis, but it has an increased risk of causing extrapyramidal symptoms such as neuroleptic malignant syndrome.

The restraints must be removed when the patient no longer poses an imminent threat to self or others and is no longer disruptive to the therapeutic setting.

PSYCHIATRIC ILLNESS IN THE ED

ED professionals often care for patients with previously diagnosed psychiatric illnesses who are ill, injured, or having a behavioral crisis. They also need to identify and manage patients with previously undiagnosed and/or undetected conditions such as suicidal ideation, depression, anxiety, psychosis, substance use and abuse, and posttraumatic stress disorder (PTSD). Psychiatric emergencies and mental health concerns account for between 2% and 5% of all pediatric hospital ED visits. Most young people who present for emergency psychiatric care are seen in general medical or adult psychiatric EDs. The experience of being in an ED is frequently difficult for children and families; the environment is noisy, crowded, and often frightening.

There are increasing concerns regarding pediatric mental health emergencies, which occur within the context of the overall crisis in pediatric ED care. First, there has been an increase in the prevalence of ED visits for psychiatric illness. This situation is complicated by a shortage of inpatient and outpatient services available for patients who need mental health care and an unfunded mandate to care for these patients in an ED setting. The National Institute of Mental Health has reported that 10% of children in the United States currently suffer from mental illness, and more than 13 million children require mental health or substance abuse services. The World Health Organization has estimated that by the year 2020, neuropsychiatric disorders will become one of the five most common causes of morbidity, mortality, and disability for children.

Suicide in the United States currently ranks as the fourth leading cause of death for 10- to 14-year-olds and the third leading cause of death for 15- to 19-year-olds, accounting for 11.3% of all deaths in the latter age group.[1] More than half of adolescents 13 to 19 years of age have suicidal thoughts, nearly 250,000 adolescents attempt suicide each year, and up to 10% of children attempt suicide sometime during their lives. Of great concern is the fact that, despite its increasing prevalence, the risk of suicidal behavior in many children and adolescents is often undetected. One study found that 83% of adolescent patients who had attempted suicide were not recognized as suicidal by their PCP.[2] Rotheram-Borus and colleagues reported that fewer than 50% of adolescents seen for suicidal behavior in the ED were ever referred for treatment; even when they were referred, compliance with treatment was low.[3] Another study revealed that only one-fifth of these children receive necessary treatment.[4]

Patients who need mental health care can disturb the routine and flow of the ED and require more resources than many medical or trauma patients. In a 2006 study, Santiago and colleagues reported that 210 patients with a median age of 14 years and requiring psychiatric evaluation spent a median of 5.7 hours in the ED. Hospital police monitored 51.9% of these patients, and 45 patients exhibited dangerous behaviors. Among children who frequently used mental health services in the ED, approximately 50% of them were seen again within 2 months of their initial visit, which suggests that patterns of recidivism are high for psychiatric patients.[5] Repeat patients are more likely to threaten to harm others; to have a diagnosis of adjustment, conduct, or oppositional disorder; and to be under the care of a child welfare agency. Repeat users were also significantly more likely than one-time patients to be less compliant with outpatient follow-up, to be admitted to the hospital, and to require more social support. These youth also have increased risk of involvement with juvenile justice; a large proportion of them have related behavioral, emotional, and cognitive disabilities and have greater difficulty remaining in residential treatment. The total proportion of children admitted to general inpatient services from the ED for mental health problems is also increasing.

PATIENT EVALUATION

The evaluation of an acute psychiatric emergency can be divided into multiple subsections. These can also be categorized as necessary information needed in making an informed decision regarding the patient's diagnosis and management in the ED.

Orienting data (gender identification, social demographics) and adequate history are used to describe the patient's general living situation and previous psychosocial history. This part of the evaluation should provide a comprehensive description of the current crisis, including apparent precipitants.

Obtaining medical history and performing the physical examination should be no different than any other ED evaluation and must happen without any anchoring bias. Psychiatric evaluation must include the patient's attention and perception, including presence or absence of auditory and visual hallucinations. One must also evaluate the patient's affect and mood, which could fluctuate between anxious, flat, tearful, and inappropriate. Speech might be non-communicative, tangential, rapid, or pressured. The patient may demonstrate abnormal behavior, including aggression, hyperactivity, withdrawal, or slowed behavior. The patient's thought content and assessment of suicidal ideation, plan of suicide, plan of homicide, or previous suicide attempts must all be very clearly documented. These have very high predictive value of future repeat events. It is important to evaluate and document the patient's impulsivity and/or inappropriate judgment because this influences disposition planning.

One always needs to remember that mental status changes could have multiple organic and medical reasons as well, and these should not be ignored.

Medical clearance of the psychiatric patient is one of the most common reasons why children and young adults with psychiatric emergencies are sent to the ED. Evaluations of such nature have multiple objectives, including determining whether a patient has an unstable medical condition or acute injury that requires immediate treatment. Many medical conditions, such as acute intoxication, head injury, endocrine emergencies, and infections, can sometimes present as acute mental status changes and need an evaluation. There are no standard lab evaluations that must be obtained to clear a psychiatric patient. However, good clinical judgment and appropriate testing might be necessary to rule out medical emergencies with patients who have an acute change in behavior.

Family evaluation, using both history and observation of the family's behavior during the ED visit, enables a physician to understand and determine the family's ability to respond to the child's distress. The emergency physician may be called upon to initiate interventions such as verbal de-escalation, physical restraint, chemical restraint, and deflection techniques (distracting from the acute situation to engage the patient by talking about things the patient enjoys). Acute psychiatric management also includes discussion with psychiatrists and interventions as recommended by them. The patient's course and management in the ED may ultimately dictate the independent disposition planning for the patient and the family.

UNIQUE FEATURES OF THE PEDIATRIC PATIENT

There are multiple challenges unique to the pediatric population in regard to psychiatric emergencies. The manifestations of suicidal behavior, depression, psychosis, schizophrenia, autism, and other pervasive developmental disorders of childhood are unique and require pointed evaluation and management.

Pediatric patients may present with dissociative disorders, which occur most commonly in females with sexual abuse as a common original trauma. Patients might present with a feeling of detachment from themselves or a feeling of being an automaton or in a dream. The emergency physician should consider the possibility of dissociative disorders in all children and adolescents who present in a confused and puzzling way. None of these children are psychotic. In fact, they are operating under an entirely different emotional process.

School refusal, school avoidance, and school phobia is another important condition with which an emergency physician should be familiar. This is usually not the initial complaint. Rather, one or more physical complaints often bring the child to the ED. By maintaining a high index of suspicion, the physician can usually detect this pattern with recurrent complaints for which no organic cause is apparent.

Another subsection of patients in the ED are children with conduct disorder. These patients engage in repetitive, socially unacceptable behavior, without evidence of medical or other psychiatric disorders. These children usually have poor adjustment at home and in the community. In addition to inconsistent limit setting by parents, separation/divorce, mental illness, and alcohol or drug abuse may also be factors. Goals for managing aggressive and disruptive children in the ED are to ensure the safety of the child, family, and staff; rule out possible medical conditions and severe psychiatric disorders before making the diagnosis of conduct disorder; and gather sufficient information to make an appropriate disposition.

Many mental health screening tools have been developed or tested in the ED setting. Although not validated in general ED populations, they have the potential to improve ED mental health screening. One example is an abbreviated version of the Home, Education/School, Activities, Drugs, Depression, Sexuality, Suicide, Safety (HEADDSSS) tool for adolescent psychosocial assessment, which was adapted for and tested in an ED. The Home, Education, Activities and Peers, Drugs and Alcohol, Suicidality, Emotions and Behaviors, Discharge Resources (HEADS-ED) tool was found to be reliable and accurate, with good concurrent and predictive validity for future psychiatric evaluation and hospitalization. The Columbia Protocol, also known as the Columbia-Suicide Severity Rating Scale (C-SSRS), supports suicide risk assessment through a series of simple, plain-language questions that anyone can ask. The answers help users identify whether someone is at risk for suicide, assess the severity and immediacy of that risk, and gauge the level of support that the person needs.

The unique social demographics, physiologic needs, and emotional aspect of treating a pediatric patient make it challenging but rewarding nonetheless.

CASE RESOLUTION

Thirty minutes after you gave him the midazolam, the patient calmed down and was able to articulate that he would not try to harm himself or anybody around him. The restraints were promptly removed, and he was monitored. When you spoke to him, he told you that when the staff had attempted to do first aid it reminded him how he had been attacked by his biological father a few years ago, and he completely lost control. He was remorseful and cried while hugging his mother.

KEY POINTS TO REMEMBER

- In the last few years, the number of pediatric patients coming to the ED for mental health evaluation and assessment has increased dramatically.
- Unique aspects of their care include social demographics and assessment, family history, presenting symptoms, and risk factors.

. Unlike other patients, pediatric patients can be de-escalated by verbal methods, by distraction, by deflection, and sometimes by appropriately working with families at bedside.

References
1. American College of Emergency Physicians. Pediatric mental health emergencies in the emergency medical services system. *Ann Emerg Med*. 2006;48(4):484–486.
2. American Academy of Pediatrics, Committee on Pediatric Emergency Medicine; American College of Emergency Physicians, Pediatric Emergency Medicine Committee. Pediatric mental health emergencies in the emergency medical services system. *Pediatrics*. 2006;118(4):1764–1767.
3. American Academy of Pediatrics, Task Force on Adolescent Assault Victim Needs. Adolescent assault victim needs: A review of issues and a model protocol. *Pediatrics*. 1996;98(5):991–1001.
4. American Academy of Pediatrics, Committee on Pediatric Emergency Medicine. Access to pediatric emergency medical care. *Pediatrics*. 2000;105(3 pt 1):647–649.
5. American Academy of Pediatrics, Child Life Council and Committee on Hospital Care. Child life services. *Pediatrics*. 2006;118(4):1757–1763.

Further Reading
American Academy of Pediatrics, Committee on Adolescence. Achieving quality health services for adolescents. *Pediatrics*. 2008;121(6):1263–1270.
American Academy of Pediatrics, Committee on Adolescence. Care of the adolescent sexual assault victim. *Pediatrics*. 2008;122(2):462–470
American Academy of Pediatrics, Committee on Adolescence. Suicide and suicide attempts in adolescents. *Pediatrics*. 2007;120(3):669–676.

18 Things Are Not Always What They Seem

Alexandra Reinbold and Nicole McCoin

A 42-year-old male with a history of hydrocephalus status post ventriculoperitoneal shunt placement, intellectual disability, spina bifida complicated by paraplegia, and neurogenic bladder, status post suprapubic catheter is transferred to the ED with 2 days of fever and vomiting. Per EMS, the providers at his long-term care facility were concerned that he may have a recurrent UTI. Assessment reveals BP 100/60, HR 105, RR 22, SpO$_2$ 95%, and rectal temp 100.6°F. The patient is awake and alert and appears uncomfortable. He whimpers and avoids eye contact. He does not respond to any questions.

What do you do now?

COGNITIVE IMPAIRMENT, AUTISM SPECTRUM DISORDER, AND DEVELOPMENTAL DISABILITIES

The emergency physician must be thorough in the clinical approach to patients with cognitive impairment, intellectual disability, developmental and behavioral challenges, and autism spectrum disorder. The clinician must be wary of three pitfalls in the workup of these patients: (1) insufficient or inaccurate patient history, (2) cursory physical examination, and (3) failure to maintain a broad differential.

PATIENT HISTORY

If airway, breathing, and circulation are intact, the physician should take a moment to obtain a thorough history. The history will help the physician understand the patient's baseline behavior and the concerns of those accompanying the patient. A thorough history will help the physician understand the environment and interactions needed to successfully complete the remainder of the physical examination.

These patients have a broad range of social and communication skills and level of function, ranging from nonverbal to mild disabilities that are difficult to detect on first glance. Physicians risk missing a diagnosis of alteration in mental status if they make improper assumptions about the patient's baseline behavior.

The physician should obtain information from as many sources as possible to ensure that all concerns regarding the patient's history are known. Initial sources include emergency medical providers and family, friends, and caregivers accompanying the patient. However, as time allows, while still early in the patient's evaluation, the physician should seek out other family members, long-term caregivers, home health nurses, primary care physicians, previous medical records, and advance directives in order to obtain all relevant information. The physician should be wary of information that has been communicated through multiple sources and should verify its accuracy. The physician may also be able to obtain a history from the patient directly. If the patient is able to communicate verbally, the clinician should establish the patient's level of health literacy and decision-making capacity.

The physician should be mindful that these patients are at risk for the same diagnoses seen throughout the ED population. However, they are also at risk for physical and behavioral conditions more commonly associated with or unique to their underlying disability. Therefore, the physician should maintain a broad differential, avoid anchoring bias, and ask both routine and unique historical questions that will establish an appropriate differential. The physician should focus on topics such as history of trauma; deviation from baseline function and activity; change in or compliance with medication regimen; medical devices present; dislodgement or malfunction of medical devices; fever or other vital sign abnormalities; increased secretions; choking episodes; changes in home ventilator settings or oxygen requirements; change in oral intake or tolerance of tube feeds; change in the appearance of the abdomen; change in appearance or quantity of urine; change in bowel habits; presence of seizure; new skin eruptions or breakdown; and bleeding diatheses.

Each of these patients may require a specialized approach to complete a full assessment. Those who know the patient best often identify the most effective strategies to interact with the patient and should be used to provide comfort. Patients may exhibit heightened emotions and responses to the new environment, particularly if they are in pain or enduring procedures.

In particular, patients with autism spectrum disorders prefer predictable environments and routine. They have a tendency toward sensory hypersensitivity and associated aggressive self-protection in response to overly stimulating situations. The clinician should ask caregivers if there are specific types of stimulation to avoid and try to prevent interactions that may extinguish trust. Efforts should be made to limit unnecessary stimulation, including auditory stimuli (e.g., monitor and pump alarms), visual stimuli (e.g., bright lights), and tactile stimuli. Physicians, nurses, and staff should rehearse "interventions" that are new to the patient with mockup items. When the patient is cooperative, they should use reward or positive verbal reinforcement. The physician should try to limit the number of involved providers with whom the patient will interact. However, in the pediatric population, child life specialists are an excellent resource and should be engaged to assist with coping and distraction methods.

In certain cases involving this patient population, coping and distraction methods fail to provide a situation in which the physician can obtain a thorough and timely exam or perform a necessary procedure. If the situation escalates and the patient or others are at high risk of physical or psychological harm, the physician should use chemical or physical restraints. These should be used only after less restrictive methods have been attempted. Warning signs for an escalating situation may include behaviors such as rocking, yelling, pacing, and increasing frequency of repetitive movements.

PHYSICAL EXAMINATION

Initial evaluation of the patient should always begin with an assessment of airway, breathing, and circulation, and the physician should address such concerns immediately. If the physician determines that the patient has altered mental status, a blood glucose should be obtained. The physician should pay careful attention to vital signs, as they provide objective data in a clinical situation where there may be limited subjective data. If there is concern for instability in vital signs, placement of supplemental oxygen, initiation of intravenous access, cardiopulmonary monitoring, and performance of a 12-lead EKG should occur as dictated by the particular vital sign abnormalities and concerns that are present.

The physician should proceed with a head-to-toe physical examination that focuses thorough attention on each organ system. In this specific scenario where the patient may be unable to effectively communicate a complete account of all of the symptoms and signs that he/she has been experiencing, the physician must be wary of overlooking a physical examination finding that may be a significant clue in determining the diagnosis.

The physician should evaluate medical devices present and assess for sources of infection or malfunction. The physician should palpate the scalp to assess for the presence of ventricular shunts and inspect the skin for any changes overlying the shunt. Particular attention should be paid to airway devices. Patients may have poor head control and require airway repositioning or adjuncts to assist with improvement in airway mechanics. Patients with a tracheostomy may also benefit from thorough suctioning, as they are often at higher risk for mucus plugging. Feeding tubes may become infected or may clog or become dislodged. Stomas and indwelling catheters should be evaluated for infection or malfunction. The physician should also assess peripheral and central lines to determine if there is any surrounding erythema, swelling, bleeding, or drainage.

Other important foci of the physical exam may include (but are not limited to) pupil size and reactivity; intraoral inspection; appearance of mucous membranes; neck mobility; regularity of cardiac rhythm; assessment of distal pulses; character of breath sounds; abdominal tenderness and presence of distention; bowel sounds; mental status changes from baseline; extremity motor exam; bony deformity or tenderness; skin eruptions; skin ecchymoses, abrasions, or lacerations; skin breakdown (including evaluating the back of the patient); and a psychiatric assessment focusing on new behaviors and change in mood. A chaperoned genitourinary exam may also be necessary, if indicated by the history, to assess skin for infection or breakdown, to assess for the presence of discharge or foreign body, and to evaluate for masses.

DIFFERENTIAL DIAGNOSIS

The physician must consider a broad differential given the possibility that communication regarding the history and performance of the physical exam is often not straightforward. The clinician should entertain both common diagnoses and those that are unique to this patient population.

Particular diagnoses to consider are medical device complications; odontogenic infections, pneumonia, urinary tract infections, and cellulitis; bowel obstructions and volvulus; seizure; foreign body; and polypharmacy. Changes in mental status or abnormal new movements could be hinting at either underlying infection or seizure disorder, although changes in mental status in those who are nonverbal could be brought about by many of these aforementioned diagnoses.

The physician should consider the possibility of abuse even if the chief complaint does not suggest it. These patients are at higher risk of abuse than the general population due to the high physical, economic, social, and emotional demands placed on their caregivers.

LABORATORY AND RADIOGRAPHIC EVALUATION

A broad workup is often necessary in these patients due to the communication barriers discussed. The physician should have a low threshold for obtaining basic laboratory studies, including complete metabolic panel (including hepatic panel), CBC with differential, urinalysis, and chest x-ray. The clinician should obtain a 12-lead EKG if the patient shows HR or BP abnormalities. The EKG will also reveal clues regarding other entities, including ongoing metabolic processes, medication effect or ingestion, or acute coronary syndrome. Other laboratory and radiographic studies will be dictated by the clinician's suspicion for a particular diagnosis. The provider should maintain a low threshold to pursue a broad infectious workup with blood and urine cultures, lactate, other markers of infection (e.g., C-reactive protein, erythrocyte sedimentation rate), and, if appropriate, lumbar puncture, as infection can have diverse presentations; obtain non-contrast head CT, especially for changes in mental status or activity, presence of ventricular shunts, or if there is a concern for trauma; maintain a low threshold for further radiographic studies if there are concerns about medical devices, trauma (e.g., extremity plain radiography), or potential intra-abdominal catastrophe (e.g., kidneys, ureters, and bladder [KUB] x-ray or abdominal CT); and consider broadening the workup significantly to include medication levels, urine drug screen, and non-contrast head CT in patients with altered mental status. Lastly, as these patients advance in age, the physician should be mindful that "common things are common," such as acute coronary syndrome and stroke, and the corresponding laboratory and radiographic workups (e.g., troponin) should be ordered when there is a suspicion for these diagnoses.

It is imperative to err on the side of ordering imaging or additional lab work when you might otherwise be willing to participate in shared decision-making with the patient and opt for close monitoring of symptoms, as these patients are often unable to adhere to "strict return precautions" or to self-monitor for symptoms.

MANAGEMENT

Management will be based on the diagnosis. The physician should have a low threshold for ordering empiric antibiotics if an infectious cause is in the differential. Physicians should follow the standard of care at each institution when repositioning or replacing medical devices and obtaining confirmatory studies to document appropriate device positioning. In general, there should be a low threshold to obtain a confirmatory study for repositioning or replacement of a device. Patients with abnormal vital signs should not be discharged. If there is concern that an underlying diagnosis has not yet been elucidated, the physician should consider admitting the patient for further workup. If there is any concern that the patient's situation upon discharge is such that he/she could not be monitored closely or given the indicated treatments, the physician should admit the patient. The physician should be cautious during disposition planning. Missed or delayed diagnoses are not uncommon in this patient population.

If the physician plans for the patient to be discharged, due to the high prevalence of comorbid behavioral health conditions, consider involving psychiatric services, social work, and case management. Thorough discharge instructions are essential as the patient's ability to keep track of his/her history may be limited and caregivers might not be present and will appreciate a written summary of the plan and any changes to the patient's routine and medications.

CASE RESOLUTION

The patient would not engage in conversation after several attempts by physicians. He was febrile, tachycardic, and hypotensive. Nurses placed the patient on cardiopulmonary monitoring, established two large-bore IVs (with additional aid at the bedside to calm the patient during placement), and administered a 1-L bolus of lactated Ringer's fluid and 1 g rectal acetaminophen. At this point, physicians were considering an infectious source, particularly a UTI, given the history provided by EMS. Fortunately, however, the name of the patient's long-term care facility was written on his gown. The physician contacted the nurse at the facility, who stated that the patient usually was more communicative and was able to answer simple questions and indicate when and where he had pain at baseline. The patient had stated that he had abdominal pain over the past 4 days. He also had not had a bowel movement over the same time period. Physicians performed a thorough physical exam and noted a distended and firm abdomen. The patient appeared uncomfortable with palpation. Bowel sounds were decreased. Laboratory and radiographic studies were performed, searching primarily for an infectious source, and KUB imaging of the abdomen was initially obtained at the bedside with plans to move to CT if needed. This

KUB demonstrated a sigmoid volvulus. The patient was admitted for further management of his volvulus.

This case highlights a presentation that could have been attributed to a UTI, but, due to a thorough history, comprehensive physical examination, and a broad differential, the correct diagnosis of volvulus was established.

KEY POINTS TO REMEMBER

· Patients with cognitive impairment and behavioral complaints pose unique challenges to physicians due to communication barriers and an extended differential diagnosis that includes diagnoses common to the general population as well as those unique to this patient population.

· Unique diagnoses to keep in the differential for these patients include medical device complication or failure; infection; intra-abdominal catastrophe; seizure and other acute neurologic events; presence of foreign bodies; and polypharmacy.

· The physician should use caution during disposition planning. Missed or delayed diagnoses are not uncommon.

Further Reading

Abramo T, Porter NW, Selby ST. The child with special healthcare needs. In: Tintinalli JE, Ma O, Yealy DM, et al., eds. *Tintinalli's Emergency Medicine: A Comprehensive Study Guide*. 9th ed. New York: McGraw-Hill Education; 2020.

Durbin A, Balogh R, Lin E, et al. Emergency department use: Common presenting issues and continuity of care for individuals with and without intellectual and developmental disabilities. *J Autism Dev Disord*. 2018;48:3542–3550. https://doi.org/10.1007/s10803-018-3615-9

Iannuzzi DA, Cheng ER, Broder-Fingert S, et al. Brief report: Emergency department utilization by individuals with autism. *J Autism Dev Disord*. 2015;45:1096–1102. https://doi.org/10.1007/s10803-014-2251-2

Vohra R, Madhavan S, Sambamoorthi U. Emergency department use among adults with autism spectrum disorders (ASD). *J Autism Dev Disord*. 2016;46(4):1441–1454. doi:10.1007/s10803-015-2692-2

Wilson CF, Strope GL, Wood JW. Acute evaluation of the child with special healthcare needs. *Pediatr Emerg Med Rep*. 2008;13:69.

19 Just Another Case of Gastro

Diane L. Gorgas

A 15-year-old girl, A.R., presents with profound weakness. This began 2 days ago with complaints of feeling fatigued and weak "like my arms and legs don't work right." The day prior to this, her mother noted that she spent "all day at the gym training for a race." Over the last 12 hours, she has refused to get out of bed and has had minimal oral intake and minimal urine output. On further questioning, the mother states that A.R. has occasionally dabbled in cannabinoid use, "as do most of the kids at her high school." A.R. reports some mild diffuse abdominal pain and lightheadedness, in addition to the weakness. Physical exam reveals HR 95, BP 100/60, RR 20, temp 37°C, SpO$_2$ 95%. Well-groomed adolescent. Height 5'5", weight 170 lbs (77 kg). In no apparent distress. Mucous membranes are dry, and her teeth are in poor condition. There is ill-defined, nontender swelling over her face, bilaterally. Lungs: Few scattered rhonchi throughout. Abd: Diminished bowels sounds throughout. Soft, mild mid-epigastric tenderness, no peritoneal signs. Skin: Poor skin turgor. Bilateral 1+ pedal edema noted. Neuro: Diffuse weakness. Deep tendon reflexes diminished throughout.

What do you do now?

BULIMIA NERVOSA

The physical exam findings, coupled with borderline low BP, high HR, and slightly low SpO_2, in a young, otherwise healthy woman, should warrant laboratory evaluation. Her laboratory exam showed severe hypokalemia (K 2.0) in association with a contraction alkalosis, with an elevated BUN of 40 and creatinine of 0.9 mg/dL. Lipase and LFTs were normal, and her CBC was unremarkable, with the exception of a slightly elevated Hgb at 15.5. Her EKG is shown in Figure 19.1.

Medically, the immediate issues are to address the patient's profound hypokalemia, hypochloremia, and metabolic alkalosis, as well as signs of volume contraction. IV hydration with potassium supplementation is critical but should be administered under strict guidelines to avoid aggressive replacement, with cardiac monitoring in place.

Most notably, the patient's laboratory work shows a profound hypokalemic, hypochloremic metabolic acidosis. These metabolic disturbances are consistent with prolonged, uncontrolled emesis. Although cannabis-associated cyclic vomiting syndrome is a reasonable first thought in this patient, a urine drug screen showing no recent cannabinoid exposure essentially rules out this diagnosis, and a negative pregnancy test rules out hyperemesis gravidarum. The patient's history of aggressively working out

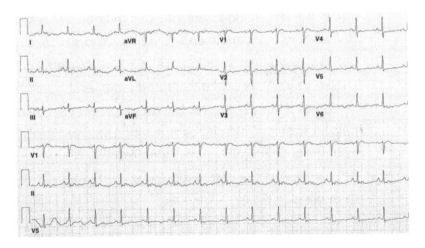

FIGURE 19.1 A.R.'s EKG

may initially point the clinician toward rhabdomyolysis as a diagnosis, but this can easily be ruled out given a normal creatinine kinase level and urine, which shows no myoglobin in the face of a normal creatinine.

There are some additional clues on her physical exam that point to bulimia nervosa (aka bulimia) as an alternative diagnosis. The cutaneous changes (Figure 19.2) on the dorsum of her right hand are consistent with Russell's sign: callus buildup as a result of repeated self-induced vomiting over long periods of time. Additionally, her generally poor dentition, in a patient who is otherwise well groomed, may speak to unintentional, longstanding dentin injury as seen with repetitive purging behavior. The negative urine drug screen should move the clinician away from a diagnosis of cannabinoid-associated cyclic vomiting and toward obtaining a more detailed eating history to help anchor a suspicion of bulimia.

A.R. shows some other physical findings suggestive of binge/purge eating. Specifically, she has parotid gland swelling, as noted with slight swelling over her lateral lower face. Salivary gland hyperstimulation from repeated self-induced emesis may also be seen with submandibular salivary gland

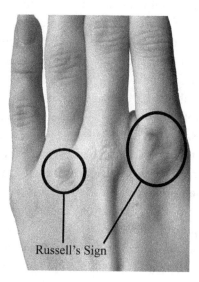

Russell's Sign

FIGURE 19.2 Russell's sign

Source: Kyukyusha. Russell's sign on the knuckles of the index and ring fingers. Wikimedia. https://commons.wikimedia.org/w/index.php?curid=5053797

enlargement. Abnormal findings in the mouth and oropharynx include (1) bruises or lacerations of the posterior oropharynx as a consequence of self-induced vomiting by fingers or other instruments to precipitate a gag reflex; (2) pyorrhea or other gum disorders; and (3) dentin loss leading to dental caries and poor dentition, particularly on the lingual surface of the teeth. Other physical findings include muscle cramping or tetany associated with hypocalcemia, and evidence of dehydration. A.R.'s weight is not abnormal for a patient with early stage bulimia, and these patients may present with either low, normal, or high BMIs.

Laboratory abnormalities associated with binge/purge eating disorders are, as classically seen here, hypokalemic, hypochloremic metabolic alkalosis; hypovolemia; and a hypokalemic myopathy (including cardiomyopathy). Other presentations can have decreased potassium secondary to diarrhea and renal losses; metabolic acidosis with spurious normal potassium; hypokalemic nephropathy; and laxative-associated laboratory abnormalities, including hypocalcemia, hypomagnesemia, and hypophosphatemia.

The prevalence of bulimia varies between boys and girls (1% for boys and 3% to 3.5% for girls) in middle- and high-income countries. Bulimia is an exceedingly rare condition in low-income countries. The disorder has a common attribute of caloric manipulation, usually manifesting as binge eating followed by purging. Despite this most common abnormal eating pattern, patients with bulimia can also demonstrate undereating or eating normal amounts of food followed by purging. In a 1991 study, Weltzin and colleagues[1] stated that 19% of bulimics undereat, 37% eat an average or normal amount of food, and 44% overeat. Closely associated eating disorder diagnoses include binge eating disorder, which is characterized by frequent and recurrent binge eating episodes, but without the following purge.

Bulimia has a high degree of comorbidity with mood disorders (depression) and anxiety and a particularly high association with borderline personality disorder (BPD). The signs of ongoing self-injurious behavior, particularly multiple superficial linear lacerations of the nondominant forearm in various stages of healing, are frequently seen with BPD.

The mainstay of therapy for patients with bulimia is to restore volume and electrolyte balance and to begin to regulate steady, predictable caloric sources. Cognitive behavioral therapy is the anchor for treatment. Antidepressants (particularly selective serotonin reuptake inhibitors [SSRIs] and tricyclic antidepressants) have shown modest benefits in acute treatment of bulimia. The rate of relapse of bulimia is high, particularly in the time soon after diagnosis and early treatment. Approximately 30% of patients relapse within 6 months. Up to 10% of patients have a chronic, indolent course of relapsing, recurrent episodic bulimia despite treatment interventions.

In addition to the medical care outlined here, the emergency physician should focus on gathering more information about dietary habits. This can be a challenge since most patients are sensitive and usually secretive about their binge eating and purging habits. An alternative to addressing A.R.'s eating habits directly may be a line of questioning with the mother present about eating disorders in the family. Between 30% and 80% of eating disorder cases have a familial component of the same. Acute decompensation, as is evidenced in A.R.'s presentation, are frequently linked to times of psychological stress, which may afford another opportunity to broach the eating pattern discussion. What cannot be emphasized enough, however, is the strong association of BPD with self-injurious behavior in this patient population. Careful examination for signs of active self-injurious behavior, such as carefully examining the entire course of both arms and both legs, is important. Although classically seen as nondominant forearm lacerations, BPD may manifest as ankle, calf, or thigh lacerations, which can easily be missed on initial examination. The immediate safety of the patient, especially with a IV potassium infusion in place, must be taken seriously. Should BPD complicate the case, it is important to know that 10% of BPD patients commit suicide in their lifetime.

CASE RESOLUTION

A.R. was admitted for potassium and fluid replacement. This was initiated with maintenance fluids with added potassium, and supplemental oral potassium was also given. The patient's weakness resolved over a 3-day period. Her caloric intake was monitored, and a sitter was provided to ensure no self-induced emesis would occur. A psychiatry consult was done on hospital day 2 and A.R. was diagnosed with bulimia and BPD. Cognitive behavioral therapy was started one on one and augmented with group therapy in an eating disorder unit. She was discharged on hospital day 5 after correction of metabolic abnormalities. Despite being enrolled in an outpatient program, A.R. had multiple relapses over the next 6 months, the first one requiring an additional hospital stay 2 months after her initial presentation. She was started on an SSRI at the time and returned again 1 week after discharge with an SSRI ingestion. She was medically stabilized from the overdose and has continued in outpatient treatment.

KEY POINTS TO REMEMBER

- Profound hypokalemia, especially in an adolescent girl when associated with metabolic alkalosis, may be associated with binge/purge eating disorder.
- The BMI is not predictive of the presence or absence of bulimia.
- Bulimia is highly associated with mood disorders (depression) and BPD, so treatment of these cases must include screening for self-injurious tendencies and suicide.
- Know the physical findings associated with bulimia (dentin destruction, Russell's sign, parotid or salivary gland swelling, pedal edema, weakness) and be sure to check for these in any young patient with vomiting.
- If an eating disorder is suspected, a family history and a social history may provide fruitful starting points for obtaining an eating history.

Reference
1. Weltzin TE, Hsu LK, Pollice C, et al. Feeding patterns in bulimia nervosa. *Biol Psychiatry*. 1991;30(11):1093–1110.

Further Reading
Bagaric M, Touyz S, Heriseanu A, et al. Are bulimia nervosa and binge eating disorder increasing? Results of a population-based study of lifetime prevalence and lifetime prevalence by age in South Australia. *Eur Eat Disord Rev*. 2020;28(3):260–268.
Bello NT, Yeomans BL. Safety of pharmacotherapy options for bulimia nervosa and binge eating disorder. *Expert Opin Drug Saf*. 2018;17(1):17–23.

Dynesen AW, Gehrt CA, Klinker SE, et al. Eating disorders: Experiences of and attitudes toward oral health and oral health behavior. *Eur J Oral Sci.* 2018;126(6):500–506.

Gibson D, Workman C, Mehler PS. Medical complications of anorexia nervosa and bulimia nervosa. *Psychiatr Clin North Am.* 2019;42(2):263–274.

He J, Cai Z, Fan X. Prevalence of binge and loss of control eating among children and adolescents with overweight and obesity: An exploratory meta-analysis. *Int J Eat Disord.* 2017;50(2):91–103.

Mehler PS, O'Melia A, Brown C, et al. Medical complications of bulimia nervosa. *Br J Hosp Med.* 2017;78(12):672–677.

Olmsted MP, MacDonald DE, McFarlane T, et al. Predictors of rapid relapse in bulimia nervosa. *Int J Eat Disord.* 2015;48(3):337–340.

20 The Refeeding Dilemma

Diane L. Gorgas

A 16-year-old girl with a history of anorexia nervosa (BMI 15) presents with a sudden onset of severe left upper quadrant abdominal pain. She relates that this began after eating boiled chicken, but she has had a history of symptoms similar to this after eating most of her meals for the last 1 to 2 weeks. She states that her pain is severe, with aching and bloating that radiates to the mid-epigastrium and also throughout her abdomen. The pain has improved in the past when she has been allowed to self-induce emesis. Vital signs: HR 49, BP 85/50, RR 28, temp 36.2°C (97.6°F), SpO_2 98%. On physical exam, her abdomen is diffusely mildly tender to palpation, but without peritoneal signs. No masses are appreciated. Her mucous membranes are dry. Laboratory testing shows Na 149, Cl 89, K 3.3, Bicarb 16, BUN 45, creat 1.1, lactate 2.4, WBC 3.1, Hgb 9.0 (Hct 28), platelets 146. The pregnancy test is negative, and her urinalysis is unremarkable.

What do you do now?

ANOREXIA NERVOSA

This case brings up two sets of management questions in a patient with anorexia nervosa (AN):

1. What are the common causes (and, conversely, life-threatening causes) of abdominal pain?
2. How should fluid management for dehydration/hypovolemic shock best be accomplished?

Patients with AN have the highest mortality among any psychiatric diagnosis, largely because of medical complications of the disease, but also because of psychiatric comorbidities. This patient population is also genetically predisposed to anxiety disorders, obsessive-compulsive disorder, and a trending toward perfectionism. Fifty percent of adolescents with AN have at least one comorbid psychiatric disorder. By definition, a BMI of 15 would classify this patient as having severe AN.

This case demonstrates the potential GI dangers associated with refeeding. Most patients with AN have an element of gastroparesis, secondary to weakened gastric motility, so initial efforts at refeeding are frequently associated with early satiety and abdominal pain or bloating. This is demonstrated in the chest radiograph obtained, which characterized by a sizeable gastric bubble. Differentiating the effects of mild gastroparesis from acute gastric dilation is important. Acute gastric dilation can cause significant abdominal pain and increases the risk of gastric perforation. An upright chest x-ray can help to rule out pneumoperitoneum from gastric rupture, or significant gastric distention from overzealous refeeding attempts (Figure 20.1). High suspicion for either gastric complication should be treated with nasogastric decompression in the ED and surgical consultation in the case of rupture.

An alternative etiology for our patient's presentation is superior mesenteric artery (SMA) syndrome. SMA syndrome is caused by extrinsic compression of the third portion of the duodenum by the SMA as a result of loss of the tissue fat pad that normally preserves the angle between the SMA and the aorta. Although either upper GI series or CT angiography can be used to diagnose SMA syndrome, CT is more sensitive and therefore the preferred test of choice, barring contraindications such as kidney injury

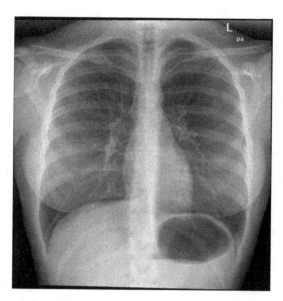

FIGURE 20.1 Chest X-ray, demonstrating large gastric bubble

from volume contraction. CT angiography will demonstrate not only the hyperacute SMA-to-aortic angle but also relative ischemia in a postprandial patient. Although surgical intervention has been explored for these patients, the mainstay of therapy is refeeding (which may require initial total parenteral nutrition) to reconstitute the fat pad and restore normal blood flow.

Other GI complications of AN and refeeding include a transient transaminitis and increased risk of hypoglycemia from depleted hepatic glucose stores. Chronic malnutrition associated with AN causes atrophy and weakness in multiple smooth muscle organ systems, including esophageal dysmotility. This can lead to choking, coughing, and increased risk of aspiration with the start of oral refeeds.

The highest risk of death in the AN patient population is from suicide and cardiac complications. A number of cardiac abnormalities associated with AN have been described in the literature, including pericardial and valvular pathology, changes in left ventricular mass and function, conduction abnormalities, bradycardia, hypotension, and dysregulation in peripheral vascular contractility. The most severe cardiac complication is sudden cardiac death, thought to be caused by chronic myocardial scarring. This was particularly true historically when syrup of ipecac was more universally available. The active ingredient in ipecac, emetine (methylcephaeline), caused permanent myocardial scarring at relatively low doses (1,250 mg cumulative dosing, when one bottle of syrup of ipecac contained 30 mg). With its restricted availability, long-term myocardial scaring has been supplanted by left ventricular atrophy and reduction in left ventricular muscle mass as the most common cardiac complication. Aggressive fluid resuscitation in these patients, even when moderately to severely dehydrated (as was demonstrated in this case by her blood pressure and lactic acidosis), should be avoided. Common vital signs and EKG abnormalities in AN include moderate bradycardia (typically less than 50 bpm) and orthostatic hypotension. QT prolongation is common but does not seem to increase the risk of torsades de pointes or sudden cardiac death. Admission to an inpatient unit with telemetry monitoring is recommended for patients with severe sinus bradycardia or junctional rhythm, marked prolongation of the corrected QT interval, or syncope. Use of echocardiography should be driven by presenting symptoms and is not routinely recommended unless syncope, dyspnea, or palpitations are present.

Other pathologic changes associated with severe malnutrition include pancytopenia (anemia, leukopenia, and neutropenia) and a blunted response to infection, with the absence of fever, even given systemic toxicity. Osteopenia and osteoporosis are common, even in adolescents after only 1 year of the diagnosis. Amenorrhea is very common in women of childbearing age afflicted with AN, but should an AN patient become pregnant, there is a high risk of obstetric and neonatal complications.

The refeeding phase for AN is associated with medical comorbidities outside of the GI system. Refeeding syndrome (RS) is one of the serious complications during AN treatment. The biggest risk factor for the development of RS is inappropriately rapid reintroduction of calories, whether orally or parenterally. This can lead to hormonal and metabolic changes, manifesting in water–electrolyte imbalances, including initial hypophosphatemia, hypokalemia, hyponatremia, hypomagnesaemia, fluid retention, vitamin deficiency, and metabolic acidosis. Wernicke's encephalopathy can occur in the refeeding phase. Contributing factors to the formation of Wernicke's include depletion of intracellular electrolytes, depletion of nutrients and vitamins, decreased basal metabolic rate, decreased renal function, decreased insulin production, and gastroparesis. Hyperphosphatemia as a result of high bone turnover, coupled with impaired renal function, is commonly seen later in the refeeding phase and should be monitored carefully.

Psychiatric treatment of AN consists of cognitive behavioral therapy (CBT) and gradual refeeding programs to improve BMI. There is no clear-cut role for antipsychotics, antidepressants, or anxiolytics in these cases, although isolated reports in the literature tout each of these.

CASE RESOLUTION

The patient was gently rehydrated with a 500-cc NS fluid bolus, and then maintenance fluids with potassium replacement were started. Her relative hypotension improved to 95/50, and her mild lactic acidosis resolved after initial fluid resuscitation. Her creatinine on recheck was 0.8 mg/dL, and she underwent a CT angiogram of the abdomen, which confirmed a diagnosis of SMA syndrome with a hyperacute angle to the SMA/aortic junction. She was admitted to a refeeding unit, a nasogastric tube was placed, and a program of around-the-clock caloric divided feeds was initiated. She tolerated the refeeding regimen well, with minimal nausea or abdominal pain, but had persistent orthostatic hypotension and bradycardia. Oral refeeding was initiated on hospital day 10 and advanced over a 2-week period. When the patient reached 80% of her predetermined daily caloric intake orally on hospital day 23, the nasogastric tube was discontinued. Her orthostatic hypotension resolved, although she remained relatively bradycardic with a resting heart rate of 55. Concomitant with her medical therapy, a comprehensive psychiatric assessment was completed and a diagnosis of obsessive-compulsive disorder was made. She was started on a selective serotonin reuptake inhibitor (SSRI) in conjunction with CBT. The patient was discharged from the inpatient refeeding program to a residential unit for an additional 2-month stay and continued in an intensive outpatient program once she returned home. Her BMI improved to 17, and her abdominal pain has not returned.

- Patients with AN can have a myriad of acute complications associated with refeeding, including aspiration pneumonia, gastroparesis, gastric rupture, and SMA syndrome.
- Physicians should have a high index of suspicion for gastric rupture and SMA syndrome in patients undergoing refeeding who have increased abdominal pain and vomiting. Do not attribute these symptoms to the psychiatric illness itself, nor to gastroparesis.
- The diagnostic study of choice for suspected SMA syndrome is CT angiography.
- The treatment of choice of SMA syndrome in a patient with moderate to severe AN is weight gain, which will generally resolve the condition.
- Volume resuscitation in dehydrated patients with active AN and signs of cardiac involvement (bradycardia) requires judicious use of fluids and careful monitoring for signs of congestive heart failure/fluid overload.

Further Reading

Bhootra K, Bhootra AR, Desai K, et al. Wernicke's encephalopathy as a part of refeeding syndrome. *J Assoc Physicians India*. 2020;68(3):80–82.

Kilbane MT, Crowley RK, Twomey PJ, et al. Anorexia nervosa with markedly high bone turnover and hyperphosphatemia during refeeding rectified by denosumab. *Osteoporos Int*. 2020;31(7):1395–1398.

Mascolo M, Trent S, Colwell C, et al. What the emergency department needs to know when caring for your patients with eating disorders. *Int J Eat Disord*. 2012;45(8):977–981.

Mitchell JE, Crow S. Medical complications of anorexia nervosa and bulimia nervosa. *Curr Opin Psychiatry*. 2006;19(4):438–443.

Trent SA, Moreira ME, Colwell CB, et al. ED management of patients with eating disorders. *Am J Emerg Med*. 2013;31(5):859–865. doi:10.1016/j.ajem.2013.02.035

Watters A, Gibson D, Dee E, et al. Superior mesenteric artery syndrome in severe anorexia nervosa: A case series. *Clin Case Rep*. 2019;8(1):185–189.

21 "Everything Hurts and I'm Weak, Doc"

Chadd K. Kraus

A 24-year-old male, Mike, presents to the ED with constant, generalized malaise and intermittent pain and weakness in both lower extremities, not associated with any exacerbating or relieving factors. The symptoms have been ongoing for "months" and he has had an extensive evaluation, including by a neurologist, MRI of the brain, and a comprehensive panel of laboratory studies. Serious neurologic, metabolic, autoimmune, and infectious etiologies have been excluded. At his PCP's recommendation, he has been seeing a psychiatrist. Mike reports that his symptoms give him great distress and he is convinced that something serious is causing the symptoms. He says, "I'm not sure I can walk. Am I going to be paralyzed, Doc?" Mike is anxious but well appearing. Vital signs are unremarkable. His physical exam is without focal findings, with normal neurologic testing of his extremities, preserved strength, brisk reflexes, intact sensation, and 5/5 strength bilaterally on his lower extremities. He ambulates in the ED with assistance and without gait abnormality.

What do you do now?

SOMATIC SYMPTOM DISORDERS

The DSM-5 classifies somatoform complaints within the broader category of somatic symptoms and related disorders. Somatic symptom disorders (SSDs) are characterized by excessive, pervasive, and disproportionate thoughts, feelings, or behaviors that are out of proportion to physical findings.

SSDs can be difficult to distinguish from the other somatic symptoms and related disorders as well as from other related conditions, making misdiagnosis common. SSD has a prevalence of 5% to 7% in the general population. For 20% to 25% of patients, SSD becomes a chronic condition, in some cases lasting for more than 5 years. Most treatment modalities are aimed at managing symptoms and coping mechanisms rather than eliminating the condition. A mainstay of treatment is long-term cognitive behavioral therapies, and in some instances adjunctive pharmacologic treatments.

SSDs present a unique challenge for the emergency physician, whose responsibility is to evaluate for, exclude, and rapidly treat immediate threats to life, limb, and vision, because these disorders are associated with disproportionate and persistent thoughts related to symptoms that may or may not be accompanied by objective medical causes. Frequently, patients with SSD present with nonspecific or vague symptoms, a history of seeking care from multiple providers for the same or similar symptoms, and chronic symptoms. The thoughts, behaviors, and symptoms associated with SSD can interfere with daily life, disrupt activities, and become debilitating. The etiology of SSD is broad and variable, and determining the cause of SSD is beyond the scope of an acute, unscheduled ED visit. It can be associated with other psychiatric conditions as well as alcohol and substance use disorders.

Extensive testing and diagnostic evaluation in patients with SSD can potentially be detrimental. Laboratory, imaging studies, and other diagnostic modalities should be limited to those necessary to exclude an emergency medical condition or a medical etiology for the symptoms. Testing can lead to incidental findings of limited to no clinical significance and will have little impact on seeking of medical care in the future.

The emergency physician in this case should, with due diligence, perform a medical screening exam and perform the minimum amount of diagnostic testing (e.g., labs, imaging). In the case presented here, the history and exam obtained do not suggest an acute, emergency medical condition as the etiology of Mike's symptoms. His symptoms are not described as acutely different or changed from baseline. The presentation is most consistent with SSD. Mike should be reassured that immediate threats to life, limb, or vision are not the etiology of his symptoms and that in the acute setting no additional testing is required. However, the emergency physician should empathetically acknowledge that what Mike is experiencing is real and has a name, SSD. It should be reinforced that the condition often manifests with physical symptoms, but he is unlikely to benefit from an extensive evaluation in the ED, particularly with the reassuring and complete workup that he has already had as an outpatient. In this case, Mike has psychiatric care already in place. If the patient has not had a psychiatric evaluation, or needs to be established with a psychiatrist or other similar professional, such arrangements for referral and follow-up should be made if possible.

CASE RESOLUTION

Mike has no clear medical or organic etiology to explain his symptoms. It should be reaffirmed that he does not require hospitalization and that his symptoms might be reduced in frequency and severity by continued outpatient management. He should be strongly encouraged to continue to attend scheduled follow-up appointments with his PCP for ongoing symptom management. It could also be recommended that Mike keep a diary of his symptoms and the circumstances surrounding them to discuss with his PCP and psychiatrist when he has follow-up appointments.

If possible and feasible, the emergency physician should make a reasonable attempt to communicate with the Mike's PCP about the ED visit, particularly because many patients with SSD will seek care in multiple settings from multiple physicians and other healthcare providers. A comprehensive approach to SSDs is fundamental to successful management of the condition. This approach requires ongoing, multidisciplinary engagement to provide the patient with frequent, regular outpatient visits, cognitive behavioral and mindfulness therapies, and in some cases pharmacologic treatments.

Finally, and with the permission of the patient, other resources, such as family and friends, could be engaged to provide additional support to the patient.

KEY POINTS TO REMEMBER

- SSD is a diagnostic challenge for the emergency physician.
- ED evaluation should include only the diagnostic testing needed to exclude an emergency medical condition.
- Treatment requires an ongoing, multidisciplinary approach with behavioral and mindfulness therapies, and in some cases pharmacologic treatments.

Further Reading

American Psychiatric Association. *Diagnostic and Statistical Manual of Mental Disorders.* 5th ed. Washington, DC: American Psychiatric Association; 2013.

Croicu C, Chwastiak L, Katon W. Approach to the patient with multiple somatic symptoms. *Med Clin North Am.* 2014;98(5):1079–1095.

Jackson JL, Kroenke K. Prevalence, impact, and prognosis of multisomatoform disorder in primary care: A 5-year follow-up study. *Psychosom Med.* 2008;70(4):430–434.

Kleinstauber M, Rief W. Somatoform and related disorders: An update. *Psychiatric Times.* 2015;32(9). https://www.psychiatrictimes.com/view/somatoform-and-related-disorders-update

Kleinstauber M, Witthoft M, Steffanowski A, et al. Pharmacological interventions for somatoform disorders in adults. *Cochrane Database Syst Rev.* 2014;11:CD010628.

Kurlansik SL, Maffei MS. Somatic symptom disorder. *Am Fam Physician.* 2016;93(1):49–54.

Rolfe A, Burton C. Reassurance after diagnostic testing with a low pretest probability of serious disease: Systematic review and meta-analysis. *JAMA Intern Med.* 2013;173(6):407–416.

Steinbrecher N, Koerber S, Frieser D, Hiller W. The prevalence of medically unexplained symptoms in primary care. *Psychosomatics.* 2011;52(3):263–271.

22 Helping the Homeless in the ED

Megan A. Panapa and Mara S. Aloi

A 45-year-old man with a history of schizophrenia presents to the ED with increasing auditory hallucinations and paranoia. He states, "The FBI implanted a mind control device in my head," and he wants it removed. He denies any attempts to take the device out himself but states that if it is not removed soon, he will "rip it out." He denies any suicidal ideation or homicidal ideation but reports he will do what he has to do in order to protect himself from the FBI. He has not taken any medications since they were stolen a month ago. The patient has a history of repeated visits over the last 5 years for alcohol intoxication, leaving prior to completion of medical care after receiving food, and occasional involuntary psychiatric admissions for suicidal command hallucinations. The patient is not welcome at the nearby shelters, given past behavioral issues, and states he lives in the city park across the street from the hospital. There are notes of the patient becoming aggressive when his demands are not met.

What do you do now?

HOMELESSNESS

It is estimated that 2.3 to 3.5 million Americans experience homelessness annually. Adults with serious mental illness, including the spectrum of schizophrenia and severe subsets of bipolar disease and depression, have a 25% to 50% increase in their risk of homelessness over their lifetime, which is 20 times higher than the general population.[1] Despite the prevalence of mental health issues in the homeless population, their contact with mental health services is generally nonexistent or at best sporadic. In addition to the burden of serious mental illness, homeless people have a very high prevalence of comorbidities, including substance use disorders and health conditions such as diabetes and heart disease. These contribute to the increased mortality in this population. Homelessness is associated with a much higher mortality risk, with a 9-fold increase in 25- to 44-year-old people and a 4.5-fold higher mortality rate in 45- to 64-year-old people when compared to the general population.[2] Additionally, regardless of housing status, patients with serious mental illness die approximately 25 years earlier than those without mental illness.[1]

It is clear that serious mental illness and homelessness are associated with significant morbidity and mortality, and we must attempt to reduce this burden. The ED has a critical role in the care of these patients as it is often their primary contact with healthcare services.

APPROACH TO PATIENT CARE

Before we can treat this patient, we have to recognize the challenges he presents to us. Encounters with homeless patients can be complicated by mutual distrust even without the amplifying effects of mental illness. Modes of interaction that protect the homeless on the street, such as exerting dominance or manipulative behaviors, can lead providers to take a guarded approach, looking for potential violence or deceit. Homeless and psychiatric patients who have been restrained, who have been held against their will, or who have had experiences of stigmatization within hospitals also approach the ED with reluctance and have a low threshold for fight-or-flight responses. Homeless mentally ill patients are disproportionately represented among patients who frequently use the ED. These repeated encounters and the difficulty in positively influencing these patients' health are distressing and dehumanizing for both providers and patients. The sense of ineffectiveness can cause compassion fatigue in providers that can translate into disengaging from or dismissing these patients. When caring for these patients, it is important to momentarily consider what biases and judgments as providers we are bringing to our conversations with them. We must recognize their behavior in the context of their daily struggles, which often focus on merely surviving another day. Additionally, understanding the historical context that created the framework for our current mental health system helps us understand the development of our patients' difficult circumstances.

HISTORY OF MENTAL HEALTH TREATMENT IN THE UNITED STATES

In the mid-1900s there was a public outcry about the inhumane treatment taking place in state mental hospitals. This led to their closure, but their replacement was never completely implemented. The Community Mental Health Act of 1963 was written with the intention of replacing these asylums with community mental health centers, but despite the optimism for the project, only half of the community mental health centers ever were built. Its failure was exacerbated by the assassination of its advocate, John F. Kennedy, and the project was never completely funded. To further disincentivize the founding of new asylums, the Institutions for Mental Disease Exclusion Act was part of the 1965 Medicaid and Medicare legislation explicitly prohibiting the federal funding of state or private hospitals that specialize in mental health care. By 2019 the number of psychiatric treatment beds plummeted to 2% to 3% of the number available in 1940 with only 14 beds for every 100,000 patient in the United States.[3]

In our country, prisons have replaced asylums. America's three largest jails serve as the country's largest psychiatric inpatient facilities, and jails across the United States hold more people with mental illness than the local inpatient units. In 2014, 20% of inmates in jails and 15% of those in state prisons had serious mental illness. Once in jail, it is difficult for patients with serious mental illness to follow or understand rules. The average stay for inmates at Rikers Island, the largest prison in New York City, is 42 days, while the average stay for people with mental illness is 215 days.[3]

ED TREATMENT

Despite these dismal realities, there is work being done to improve the outcome of homeless people with serious mental illness, and EDs play a critical role in these efforts. Although it is not possible for medicine to solve all of humanity's ills, emergency physicians can be advocates for these patients by reducing their burden of disease by offering excellent medical treatment, connecting these patients to homeless-specific services and resources, and providing care that is free of blame for those who face very challenging circumstances.

Among the important aspects of the medical treatment of homeless patients with mental illness is completing a psychiatric risk assessment, reinitiating psychiatric treatment while controlling agitation, ruling out organic causes of their psychiatric symptoms, and treating their withdrawal from substances while they await treatment. The psychiatric risk assessment is not different for the homeless population but is challenged by the interpretation of "unable to care for self." This is not a complete discussion of this subject, but these assessments will be dependent on the judgment of the provider and will be informed by the state laws, and perhaps a discussion with a consulting psychiatrist.

These patients are at high risk of agitation that can put you and your staff's safety at risk. Patients with known psychosis should be restarted on their previous medication or an antipsychotic medication, hopefully prior to escalation of their symptoms. If a patient does worsen and verbal de-escalation is ineffective, chemical restraints and physical restraints should be considered. There are many options for chemical restraints, but common options include haloperidol (Haldol) 0.5 to 5 mg (with or without lorazepam 2 mg or diphenhydramine 50 mg) via any route (IM, PO, IV), or ziprasidone 10 to 20 mg IM.

Organic causes of psychosis or psychotic symptoms are broad, including a large differential for delirium and encephalopathy, which we should be careful not to dismiss as possible causes of our homeless patient's symptoms, even with a history of schizophrenia. Homeless patients are at increased risk for particular mimics of psychosis, including traumatic intracranial hemorrhage and nutritional deficiencies, because of their high level of substance abuse and the environment in which they live. An acute or chronic subdural hematoma can present as withdrawal, cognitive dysfunction, and blunted affect consistent with schizophrenic catatonia. A physical exam for signs of trauma is important for these patients but can be challenging or limited due to their mental status. Have a low threshold for head imaging in this population, especially in the setting of new-onset psychotic symptoms or if the patient is refractory to typical antipsychotics.

Nutritional deficits and malnutrition should also be a consideration for the homeless population, especially for those who live outside of shelters or have alcohol use disorder. Significant B-vitamin deficiencies, including thiamine deficiency and niacin deficiency, have been associated with this population.

Severe thiamine deficiency can cause Wernicke's encephalopathy, which is associated with ataxia, memory loss, confusion, and ocular abnormalities. Failure to diagnose this in a timely fashion causes death in 17%, and the remaining 84% of patients may have permanent brain damage.[4] The symptoms of this are usually severe short-term memory loss and hallucinations, known as Korsakoff's syndrome. It is important to consider thiamine supplementation in anyone with nutritional deficiency, cerebellar or oculomotor abnormalities, or impaired mental state or memory. This represents a large number of homeless patients with serious mental illness.

Niacin deficits traditionally have been known to cause the "three D's": dermatitis, diarrhea, and dementia; however, it is thought that dementia is better explained by the term "delirium." These symptoms rarely present together, and they present with varying levels of severity, so it can be difficult to recognize.

For our homeless patients with psychiatric symptoms and alcoholism, niacin and thiamine supplementation should be considered. Laboratory testing is not helpful in an ED setting. Therefore, supplementation should happen empirically. If there is concern for Wernicke's encephalopathy, IV doses of thiamine 500 mg three times a day are recommended as the oral absorption of thiamine is variable. This should be paired with supplementation of nicotinamide at least 300 mg PO or 100 mg daily IV.

Both homelessness and psychiatric illness are associated with substance abuse disorder. One-third of the approximately 100 million homeless people in the world are alcohol dependent and, in one study conducted in Boston, overdose contributed to a third of deaths of their homeless population.[2] This is not a complete discussion about the treatment of addiction, but in the treatment of these patients who are often boarding in the ED for a long period of time, we should be monitoring for the symptoms of withdrawal and treating for it. For patients who are being discharged, consider initiating addiction treatment in the ED as well as providing naloxone for those who are opioid dependent. These patients should be also connected with outpatient resources for addiction treatment.

Our homeless psychiatric patients also benefit from services that are specifically for the homeless or frequent ED users, such as intensive case management programs and "housing first" interventions. "Housing first" programs are based on a concept of providing permanent housing and wraparound support services to undomiciled patients upon discharge from a healthcare facility. Such programs do not have the preconditions for housing that many traditional housing programs do, such as requirements for sobriety or participation in substance abuse treatment programs. Instead, these programs are based on the idea that without the stability of a home, people find it very difficult to attend to their medical or psychiatric needs. There have been various studies of these programs that have shown increased use of outpatient services, decreased ED visits, decreased healthcare costs, and even decreased need for substance abuse treatment. Intensive case management has shown similar findings. One study compared a comprehensive "housing first" program plus intensive case management with intensive case management alone. It demonstrated that for those with severe mental illness or substance use, comprehensive services improved outcomes such as mental health symptoms, substance use, and quality of life, but for those with lower severity, case management alone was enough to improve outcomes.[5] Being knowledgeable about the services that can be offered to your patients and, if possible, championing the generation of further programs would benefit these patients greatly. Engaging your ED social worker can also be a high-yield step.

CASE RESOLUTION

The patient was not deemed to be a risk to himself or others and did not require admission for emergency psychiatric stabilization. He refused to be restarted on the antipsychotic medication regimen he was previously on but did agree to speak with the ED social worker about a local "housing first" program. He chose a housing facility in close proximity to his aunt, with whom he had a close relationship. A psychiatric social worker and crisis management team were assigned to him and were able to assess him frequently, ultimately getting him back on medical therapy and into group sessions. The frequency of his ED visits drastically decreased.

KEY POINTS TO REMEMBER

- Homelessness and serious mental illness are associated with high mortality.
- These healthcare encounters can be challenging for both providers and patients. Try to be aware of the judgments and bias we bring to these conversations.
- There is a historical context for the current circumstances for those with serious mental illness that can help us understand their circumstances.
- Look for mimics of psychiatric disease such as traumatic intracranial hemorrhage and nutritional deficiencies.
- Treat substance abuse and its complications in the ED.
- Connect your patients to "housing first" programs and intensive case management. If your community doesn't have these programs, consider starting them.

References

1. Bauer LK, Baggett TP, Stern TA, et al. Caring for homeless persons with serious mental illness in general hospitals. *Psychosomatics*. 2013;54(1):14–21. doi:10.1016/j.psym.2012.10.004
2. Baggett TP, Hwang SW, O'Connell JJ, et al. Mortality among homeless adults in Boston: Shifts in causes of death over a 15-year period. *JAMA Intern Med*. 2013;173(3):189–195. doi:10.1001/jamainternmed.2013.1604

3. Rosenberg KP. *Bedlam: An Intimate Journey into America's Mental Health Crisis.* 1st ed. New York: Avery; 2019.
4. Dhir S, Tarasenko M, Napoli E, et al. Neurological, psychiatric, and biochemical aspects of thiamine deficiency in children and adults. *Front Psychiatry.* 2019;10:207. doi:10.3389/fpsyt.2019.00207
5. Clark C, Rich AR. Outcomes of homeless adults with mental illness in a housing program and in case management only. *Psychiatr Serv.* 2003;54(1):78-83. doi:10.1176/appi.ps.54.1.78.

Further Reading

Braslow JT, Messac L. Medicalization and demedicalization: A gravely disabled homeless man with psychiatric illness. *N Engl J Med.* 2018;379(20):1885–1888. doi:10.1056/NEJMp1811623

Henry M, Watt R, Mahathey A, et al. The 2019 Annual Homeless Assessment Report (AHAR) to Congress. https://www.huduser.gov/portal/sites/default/files/pdf/2019-AHAR-Part-1.pdf

O'Carroll A, Wainwright D. Making sense of street chaos: An ethnographic exploration of homeless people's health service utilization. *Int J Equity Health.* 2019;18(1):113. doi:10.1186/s12939-019-1002-6.

Torrey EF. *American Psychosis.* New York: Oxford University Press; 2013.

Suicidal Ideation with Vague and Contradicting History

Melinda Nguyen and Mohamad Moussa

A 40-year-old male presents to the ED on a cold winter's evening with the complaint of suicidal ideation. In addition to suicidal ideation, the patient admits to depression. He adds that he has thoughts of jumping off a building, and if he is discharged, he will undoubtedly end his life. The patient continues to endorse suicidal ideation and depression, and without further questioning, adds that he has the sudden onset of auditory hallucinations of a female's voice in a language he did not recognize. He is quick to agree with follow-up questions but when pressed for further details, they are vague and/or extremely exaggerated. Throughout the examination, the patient repeatedly asks for food. On initial examination the patient is noted to be thin and unkempt, with poor dentition. His speech is unremarkable and he has normal eye contact. He is cooperative, with a logical thought process. His nurse notes that the patient has been sleeping comfortably and eating well.

What do you do now?

MALINGERING

Diagnosis of Malingering

The most common differential diagnoses when a patient presents to the ED with psychiatric symptoms include psychosis due to an underlying health condition, medications, or drug use. Labs ordered should include a CBC, comprehensive metabolic panel, urinalysis, alcohol screen, and urine drug screen. After the results are returned, if all values are found to be within normal limits, and there is no substance present in the system that could explain an acute response, one can rule out symptoms caused by medication or drug use.

The next step in care is to further evaluate the patient for underlying mental illness. The ED social worker, if available, can provide service development for patients who are afflicted with mental illness, those who exhibit evidence of social dysfunction, those who are suffering from inhospitable home environments, or those in danger of deliberate self-harm. If the patient continues to endorse suicidal ideation to the social worker, then the patient must speak with psychiatry for further action. In the case presented, the psychiatrist notices a discrepancy between the patient's history and physical exam. By prolonging the interview, asking rapid-fire questions, and leading the patient during the examination, inconsistencies or contradictions suggesting malingering as a root cause of the patient's chief complaint surfaced. The psychiatrist began to suspect malingering through diagnosis of exclusion.

Though the psychiatrist may feel that the patient is malingering and is safe for discharge, the emergency medicine physician may feel uncomfortable sending the patient away if he continues to endorse suicidal ideation. In addition, extreme caution must be used when labeling a patient as a malingerer, as a false characterization can result in distrust in health professionals or, worse, missing a potentially critical diagnosis.

Given that the prevalence of suspicion of malingering in patients who present to the ED with behavior consistent with malingering is 33%, with the prevalence of *strong* suspicion of malingering in 20% of patients,[1] it is vital to be able to recognize the signs of malingering to optimize patient care and provide patients with alternative actions.

Tests for Malingering

Two tests that can be performed at bedside that are helpful in detecting malingering are the Miller Forensic Assessment of Systems Test (M-FAST) and the Coin in the Hand Test (CIH test).

The M-FAST is a 25-item structured interview that takes approximately 5 to 10 minutes to administer. It includes items developed from seven strategies found previously to differentiate malingerers from honest responders. These strategies include unusual hallucinations (reported vs. observed), extreme symptomatology, rare combinations, negative image, unusual symptom course, and suggestibility. The items for the instrument were created based on methods of questioning that have been effective in identifying overreporters previously. The items are summed to produce a total score. A total score of 6 or more indicates possible malingering. A meta-analysis of the M-FAST found that the total score seems to be useful in detecting the overreporting involved in malingering. Nevertheless, any positive results should be followed by additional assessment to prevent mislabeling patients as malingerers, which could have serious ramifications.[2]

The CIH test was developed to detect the presence of malingering in patients who are suspected of simulating poor memory performance. In this task, a coin is held in either the left or right hand of the presenter, and the patient is given 2 seconds to look at the coin and memorize which hand is holding it. Then the patient is told to close his eyes and count down from 10. When the patient has finished counting, he is asked to open his eyes and point to the clenched fist that he believes holds the coin. This test is repeated 10 times and the provider gives feedback on whether the answer is accurate or inaccurate. A study comparing patients with a neurologic disorder to suspected malingerers found that in patients with a neurologic disorder, there is no difference in performance by a control group. In contrast, the suspected malingerers usually and deliberately achieved, at best, at the chance level. This illustrates how suspected malingerers incorrectly believe that patients who endorse psychological or mood symptoms also endorse cognitive impairment.[3]

It is likely that no single test in itself will be sufficient to prove the presence of malingering, and additional tests, including the Minnesota Multiphasic Personality Inventory, the Structured Interview of Reported Symptoms, the Rey 15-item visual memory test, and the symptom validity test, among others, can also be used in conjunction with the M-FAST and the CIH test to screen for malingering. These results can be used to formulate a more comprehensive clinical impression. However, before the physician can declare that the patient is indeed exaggerating his/her symptoms and prepare to discharge the patient, it is essential to appreciate the latent circumstances that motivate the patient to feign illness. Therefore, the reasons behind the actions of the malingering patient must be understood.

Understanding the Malingering Patient

Malingering itself is not designated as a mental illness. It is defined by the DSM as the intentional production of false or grossly exaggerated physical or psychological symptoms, motivated by external incentives.

There are three main types of malingerers who seek care in the ED. The first hopes to gain goods and services, such as a warm bed and food or prescriptions for opiates or benzodiazepines to fuel an addiction. The second type of malingerer uses the ED to avoid the state of affairs in his/her life, such as seeking refuge from domestic violence or avoiding a court date. The last type of malingerer may be seeking care as part of a plan to extract a medical liability settlement from the hospital. This type of patient is less common but may be the most pernicious.

Malingering can also be a symptom of or be confused with another mental illness, such as conversion disorder or factitious disorder. It is a challenge to differentiate malingering from conversion disorder. Conversion disorder is characterized by neurologic symptoms such as weakness, nonepileptic seizure, and weakness. These symptoms are inconsistent with neurologic disease but are real and cause distress and/or impair normal social interactions. The feigning of symptoms is unintentional and often preceded by stressors or conflict.

Factitious disorder is also often mistaken for malingering. A patient with a factitious disorder will intentionally feign an illness, with no obvious external reward other than to be perceived as handicapped, ill, or wounded. In contrast, the malingering patient has a goal to achieve. Since both involve fabricated symptoms and similar general behavior, it is difficult to differentiate between them. Therefore, it is important to pay attention to possible motivations prompting the patient to seek care in the ED.

Gathering additional information from those who have interacted with the patient, such as nurses, paramedics, police, family, or friends, or gaining further insight into patterns from past medical history, can elucidate whether the case is truly an example of malingering or if the perceived symptoms are due to another psychiatric illness. The malingering patient can hope to be admitted to the hospital or he/she may be satisfied by being kept overnight where he/she is rested and fed. Either way, effective management of suspected malingering should begin with the working assumption that the patient has a legitimate need for care.

Compassionate Care

At even the faintest indication of malingering, a physician can easily write off a patient, for every bed in the ED occupied by a malingering patient means time and resources taken away from other patients who need to be seen. This directly affects other patients waiting for treatment or waiting for final results. As federal programs pay for some of the treatment received by malingerers, taxpayers can also be indirect victims of this deception. One study found that the estimated costs of malingered mental disorders for Supplemental Security Income (SSI) and Social Security Disability Insurance programs in 2011 were $20.02 billion.[4]

However, if the ED staff focuses only on the malingering and concludes that the patient's complaints are not legitimate, or at least not treatable, the staff has missed an important opportunity to help these patients. The individuals who lack shelter or food, who are facing domestic abuse, or who have a substance use disorder still need care. When malingering is suspected, the physician should communicate to the patient that people turn to the ED for help with a variety of problems, some of which can be dealt with at the hospital and some of which cannot. The patient should be informed that the physician is committed to doing everything possible to ensure that the patient's needs are met, but those needs are likely better served through services outside of the ED.

Final Thoughts

There are three possible conclusions that come from an interaction with a patient who is identified as a malingerer. The most hoped-for outcome is that after speaking with the patient and noting the inconsistencies in his/her history and symptoms, the patient will cooperate and take the opportunity to reveal the reasons why he/she has been using the sick role to be evaluated in the ED. This disclosed information can maximize the ability of hospital staff to connect the patient to the resources that he/she needs. In the second outcome, the patient may cooperate with the assessment but leave once it is clear that his/her goals will not be met. For example, if a malingering patient is demanding opioids for a headache but only alternative forms of treatment, such as trigger point injections, are being offered, he/she may choose to be discharged against medical advice. However, the most difficult outcome is the patient who fails to be honest and cooperate despite the best efforts of staff to treat him/her in a nonjudgmental way. In this case, the hospital should ensure that careful records are kept that document the genuine efforts that have been made to help the patient and his/her continued resistance to this assistance. At this point, the physician can either choose to keep the patient for overnight observation or discharge the patient home. In the case of malingering, patients with the highest degree of suspicion can be discharged rather than held for observation, which demonstrates the certainty of assessments and lack of symptoms necessitating further care. However, if there is even the smallest suggestion that the patient could be harmed by being discharged, then the more conservative action must be taken.

It is undoubtedly a challenge to recognize the signs of a malingering patient, as there is not one single pathognomonic symptom or designated test to definitively identify a malingerer. It is even more difficult addressing the patient over the concern in a non-accusing and respectful approach. Extreme caution and mindful phrasing must be exercised when confronting the patient about his/her fabricated symptoms. Ultimately, it is important to keep in mind that people with feigned illness often do need help. However, the help they need is likely found through the resources a social worker can provide, such as referrals to free clinics, shelters, safe houses, and rehabilitation centers—not in the ED.

CASE RESOLUTION

The emergency medicine physician chooses to err on the side of caution and keep the patient for a few hours for observation. He receives hot food and footie socks. After reevaluation, the patient states that his symptoms have improved and denies suicidal or homicidal ideation. The patient meets with the department social worker and is placed in a new adult homeless shelter after it is determined that the underlying cause of the visit was for external gains. A cab ride is called, and he is discharged to the new shelter.

KEY POINTS TO REMEMBER

- The most common complaint of a malingerer is suicidal ideation, as testing is based on self-reported symptoms and the consequences are potentially fatal.
- Patients with true psychosis often have to be encouraged to take medication. Malingering patients will insist that only specific medications can treat their illness.
- A malingering patient will make dependent or conditional threats if his/her demands are not met. Patients with severe psychotic thoughts generally do not have the motivation for such threats.
- Patients with mood disorders or other mental illness are not readily forthcoming with their symptoms and will only disclose details when rapport is established with the physician. Malingering patients will readily endorse symptoms, sometimes dramatically.
- When asked questions, the malingering patient may be either vague, responding with numerous "I don't know's," or be uncooperative, refusing to engage in the interview.
- Malingering patients may endorse improbable (such as both visual and auditory hallucinations) or contradicting symptoms (both depressive moods and euphoria).
- Endorsing or demonstrating both psychiatric symptoms (psychosis) and cognitive deficits (impaired memory) may be signs of malingering.

References
1. Rumschik SM, Appel JM. Malingering in the psychiatric emergency department: Prevalence, predictors, and outcomes. *Psychiatr Serv.* 2019;70(2):115–122. doi:10.1176/appi.ps.201800140

2. Detullio D, Messer SC, Kennedy TD, Millen DH. A meta-analysis of the Miller Forensic Assessment of Symptoms Test (M-FAST). *Psychol Assess.* 2019;31(11):1319–1328. doi:10.1037/pas0000753

3. Kapur N. The coin-in-the-hand test: A new "bed-side" test for the detection of malingering in patients with suspected memory disorder. *J Neurol Neurosurg Psychiatry.* 1994;57(3):385–386. doi:10.1136/jnnp.57.3.385

4. Chafetz M, Underhill J. Estimated costs of malingered disability. *Arch Clin Neuropsychol.* 2013;28(7):633–639. doi:10.1093/arclin/act038

24 Down on the Farm

Lauren E. Valyo and Mara S. Aloi

It's 5 p.m. on a hot June day, and you are working in a rural hospital in central Pennsylvania. A 22-year-old female is brought in by EMS after a syncopal episode. Her vitals on arrival are BP 104/60, HR 106, RR 18, SpO_2 99, temp 37.3°C. EMS reports that she was awake, alert, and sipping water when they arrived on scene at a local farm. According to her supervisor, who called 911, she is a foreign exchange student who took a summer internship. The agriculture team was out all day in the fields, and the patient had a 15-second syncopal episode with immediate recovery. You notice a tired but pleasant-appearing young female wearing a hijab. As you start your exam, the nurse urgently pulls you aside to speak with the patient's supervisor, who has just arrived. He tells you that he thinks this patient needs a psychiatric evaluation because "she has been working at my farm for over 2 weeks now and doesn't eat or drink anything all day long. I offer her food and drink and she refuses. She hasn't eaten in over 2 weeks! I think she is anorexic."

What do you do now?

CULTURALLY COMPETENT EMERGENCY CARE

Patients from minority groups disproportionately use the ED for many of their healthcare needs. It is known that culture and society play a large role in mental health. In some cultures, mental illness is the result of perceived supernatural causes, imbalance of "energies," or even dietary indiscretions. In addition, having a mental illness can be associated with societal stigma. Multiple studies have shown that minorities of all types are less likely to seek psychiatric help than culturally westernized Whites and are more likely to present late in the course of their disease. This is due to multiple factors, such as cultural stigma associated with psychiatric illnesses and/ or medications; socioeconomic limitations, which disproportionately affect ethnic and racial minorities; desire to see a psychiatric provider of a similar race/ethnicity and being unable to find one; and mistrust of the healthcare system.

The mandate to us as emergency providers is to deliver equitable care to all patients who come through our doors, with the added challenges of language barriers, differences in cultures, and the time and space constraints found in most busy EDs. This highlights the needs for cultural competence in order to improve the doctor–patient relationship. It requires us to understand patients' conceptualization of their disease, to elicit their explanation for their symptoms, and to devise a treatment plan that is culturally compatible for them.

As emergency physicians and not cultural anthropologists, we cannot possibly know everything about all cultures. A helpful resource is https:// www.crculturevision.com/. This is a service that healthcare providers can access when they encounter a patient from a culture with which they are not familiar, and is helpful for all cross-cultural interactions in the ED, not just psychiatric-related encounters. But outside of this site, how can you be more cognizant of bridging culture gaps in psychiatric care in the ED? The DSM-5 contains a *Cultural Formulation Interview* (CFI) section, which contains 16 questions that may be asked during a psychiatric interview to bridge culture gaps. Aspects of the CFI that are applicable to the ED include an assessment of the patient's cultural identity, cultural conceptualization of diseases, and presence of any psychosocial stressors (e.g., refugee status, wartime experience, immigration difficulties). A stressor unique to the foreign-born patient is acculturation stress or "culture shock," the temporary feeling of being overwhelmed when moving to a new setting. This should not be confused with posttraumatic stress disorder.

Consider the patient's culture and religion when performing an assessment to avoid any patient discomfort and damage to the physician–patient relationship. Some patients will not permit an exam by a healthcare provider of the opposite sex. Also be sensitive to your patient, and consider that differences in nonverbal communication may interfere with your interaction. For example, direct eye contact may be seen as somewhat aggressive by some groups. Casual touch, such as a pat on the shoulder, may be insulting to others. Extended family groups and community leaders have special importance for patients in many ethnic groups, so attempt to engage them when possible. These can be crucial to supporting patient compliance with follow-up services that are arranged in the ED.

Ideally, the assessment should be done in the patient's native language, using a trained interpreter rather than ad hoc interpreters, such as a patient's family members or friends. Vital information can be lost when using untrained interpreters, especially when discussing sensitive topics, such as sexual or substance abuse issues. Their use can lead to errors, violation of confidentiality, and poor outcomes. Children should never be used as interpreters except in emergencies. Title VI of the Civil Rights Act requires hospitals to provide interpretive services for patients with limited English proficiency. The benefits of using a trained medical interpreter include fewer communication errors, improved patient satisfaction, shorter hospital stays, and decreased readmission rates. The interpreter may also serve as a liaison, explaining the norms and behaviors of the patient's culture, especially as it relates to the patient's attitudes about illness and expectations of care. Interpreters can also explain *cultural idioms of distress*, which are ways of expressing stress that are shared among members of a certain culture. A full description of these is beyond the scope of this chapter. When conducting a patient assessment with the aid of an interpreter, address the patient directly rather than the interpreter, ask only one question at a time, and allow time at the end of the encounter to review with the patient what has been discussed, to ensure that you have received an accurate representation of the situation.

ED MANAGEMENT

First and foremost, remember that the general rules of ED psychiatry still apply. The safety of yourself and staff comes first, so patients who pose a threat to you, themselves, or others need to be chemically and/or physically restrained. If the patient is not posing an active threat, a psychiatric and medical exam must be performed. Patients who have active suicidal ideation or homicidal ideation or are unable to care for themselves and are unwilling to voluntarily receive inpatient treatment must not be allowed to leave the ED. Terminology regarding involuntary admission varies across the United States, so reference the laws in your state and take appropriate action to have the patient admitted to the hospital involuntarily, if he/she meets the criteria above.

Remember that these patients still require a full medical evaluation to rule out any serious medical comorbidities. Medical clearance requirements vary by institution as well but generally consist of a thorough physical and neurologic exam, as well as basic labs plus acetaminophen and salicylate levels, urine drug screen, and serum ethanol. Use of folk medicine is highly prevalent in patients from non-Western cultures. It is important to elicit a history of alternative treatments the patient may have received as these may be the etiology of the presenting complaint or may result in a medication interaction with any treatments offered in the ED.

The following PSYCH mnemonic may help you bridge the concept of cultural differences in a potential psychiatric patient in an appropriate manner. It may facilitate discussion of psychiatric complaints in all patients, but especially in psychiatric patients from a different cultural community:

> **P: Perception.** What is the patient's perception of what is wrong, or what concerns them? What is their perception of medical care and Western forms of treatment? For example, while insomnia might indicate underlying depression to you, the patient may be more concerned about supernatural causes, such as presence of a malevolent spiritual being, and may want that addressed first. This gives you insight into how their cultural identity may bring different concerns than your own to the forefront of their care. It also sets the stage by giving you more information about their understanding of their current condition.

S: Symptoms. What symptoms are they having, and why do they think they are having them? What do the symptoms mean to them? They may not bring up psychiatric concerns at all, and if your clinical suspicion for psychiatric illness persists, gaining a sense of the patient's perception of their illness will help you sensitively broach the topic of a psychiatric ailment during your discussion. For example, in some cultures, because of the stigma associated with mental illness, it is common for symptoms of depression to present with *solely* physical complaints such as fatigue, headache, weakness, insomnia, or lack of appetite. If you fail to empathize with their cultural perception of symptoms, you will not be able to develop rapport with them.

Y: Why. Why are they seeking treatment? What do they hope to gain? Cultural differences definitely affect the types of treatment that people may seek and the end goal they may desire. Listen to their goals; they may be different than typical Western goals of therapy. You will not accomplish success or a positive patient experience by forcing your goals on a patient who does not value them.

C: Culture. Ask culturally sensitive questions about how they feel that their life has been molded by their cultural/familial/racial experiences and influences, if relevant. Not all patients who have culturally different backgrounds than our own will find/deem culture to be a significant influence in their choices to seek mental help. If the patient does not report significant life/cultural/racial/ migration experiences to be influencing their presentation, do not pressure them for this information. Validate your patient's distress by saying things like "*I can't imagine* how difficult that must be to cope with." This is also a good time to address any concerns that the patient may have about your own culture and how it may influence the encounter. You could say, "Sometimes doctors and patients misunderstand each other because they come from different backgrounds or have different expectations. Are you concerned about this and is there anything that we can do to provide you with the care you need?"

H: Help. In response to the question above, give them culturally appropriate options to seek help. Bring in a social worker, a religious figure, or a community leader, if available and desired, to talk to the patient about options that fit best for their cultural needs and desires.

CASE RESOLUTION

This patient was not an immediate threat to staff members or herself and was not truly a psychiatric patient. You were told that she is a foreign exchange student, so you should expect that the culture of the patient, the supervisor's culture, and your own culture affected the encounter. The farmer for whom she is an intern believed that she had not eaten or drank anything in 2 weeks. You know that this was improbable since she would have shown some clinical signs of volume depletion. The patient's religion was Islam, as she was wearing a hijab. When treating this patient, it was necessary for the emergency physician to have some awareness of Islamic beliefs and rituals. The time of year was June, and depending on the year, the Islamic holy month Ramadan may have fallen in June. During Ramadan, it is Islamic practice to fast from sunrise to sunset each day, with few exceptions. At sunset, Muslims taking part in Ramadan will break their fast by drinking fluids and eating a large meal, and are able to eat or drink at any time during the night.

This patient was fasting during the day for Ramadan. She continued to sip water in the ED and even ate a few crackers, stating that in her religion, she was permitted to discontinue the fast because of health concerns. She explained her practice to her supervisor, who appeared relieved that she was not truly suffering from anorexia nervosa.

KEY POINTS TO REMEMBER

- What we as Western clinicians might consider pathologic may be acceptable in a patient's culture (e.g., spirit possession, witchcraft for healing rituals).
- Conduct the assessment in the patient's native language, using professional translators rather than untrained interpreters.
- Attempt to identify and address barriers that may prevent your patient from accessing mental health and family services.

- Screen for the use of any alternative therapies that may impact your patient's clinical presentation (i.e., side effects, interactions with prescribed agents).
- Assess for a history of trauma or immigration-related stress so that appropriate resources can be offered to the patient.
- Find out what resources are available in your institution that will aid you in caring for patients from different cultures.

Further Reading

American Psychiatric Association. *Glossary of Cultural Concepts of Distress*. https://doi.org/10.1176/appi.books.9780890425596.GlossaryofCulturalConceptsofDistress

American Psychiatric Association. Outline for Cultural Formation. In: *Diagnostic and Statistical Manual of Mental Disorders, Text revision*. 5th ed. Washington, DC: American Psychiatric Association; 2013.

Center for Substance Abuse Treatment. *Improving Cultural Competence in Treatment Improvement Protocol (TIP) Series*, No. 59. Rockville, MD: Substance Abuse and Mental Health Services Administration; 2014.

Cook Ross Inc. CultureVision. https://www.crculturevision.com/

Leseth AB. What is culturally informed psychiatry? Cultural understanding and withdrawal in the clinical encounter. *BJPsych Bull* 2015;39(4):187–190.

Lewis-Fernández R, Aggarwal NK. Culture and psychiatric diagnosis. *Adv Psychosom Med*. 2013;33:15–30.

Office of Minority Health, U.S. Department of Health and Human Services. *Think Cultural Health: A Physician's Practical Guide to Culturally Competent Care*. https://cccm.thinkculturalhealth.hhs.gov/default.asp

Office of the Surgeon General; Center for Mental Health Services. Culture Counts: The Influence of Culture and Society on Mental Health. Chapter 2 in: *Mental Health: Culture, Race, and Ethnicity: A Supplement to Mental Health: A Report of the Surgeon General*. Rockville, MD: Substance Abuse and Mental Health Services Administration; 2001. http://ncbi.nlm.nih.gov/books/NBK44249/?report=printable

25 You're Staying, Whether You Like It or Not

Chadd K. Kraus

A 26-year-old male presents to the ED in police custody after a verbal altercation with his significant other. The police report that the patient threatened to "end it all" and according to the patient's significant other, he drank "a lot of beer" throughout the day. In the ED, the patient is calm and cooperative and tells you, the emergency physician, that he "didn't really mean it" when he made the statement. He repeatedly denies overt suicidal or homicidal thoughts in the ED. The physical exam is unremarkable, he has no visible injuries, and he is calm and interactive. Vital signs are HR 88, BP 118/72, RR 16, temp 98.4°F, and SpO_2 97% on room air. A blood alcohol test shows that the patient is not legally intoxicated, and he does not clinically appear to be under the influence of alcohol or drugs. The patient's significant other is requesting to "commit" the patient for psychiatric evaluation, because she is concerned for his safety, but the patient does not think he needs to be evaluated by a psychiatrist.

What do you do now?

INVOLUNTARY COMMITMENT

Involuntary commitment, legally holding a patient for psychiatric evaluation over his/her objections or without his/her consent, presents a challenging ethical dilemma for the emergency physician. "Involuntary commitment for psychiatric conditions" is the term used in this chapter. However, involuntary commitments are known by a variety of synonymous terms, including emergency holds, 72-hour holds, emergency commitment, psychiatric hold, temporary detention order, or an emergency petition. These vary in characteristics and regulatory and legal statute on a state-by-state basis.

Suicidality is a common reason for involuntary psychiatry hold in the ED. Patients with homicidal thoughts are less common, and many of them have concomitant suicidality. There are also considerable comorbid substance and/or alcohol use disorders among patients with psychiatric conditions, further complicating involuntary commitment. In some cases, a patient clearly poses a risk of harm to himself/herself and is unwilling to be hospitalized despite requiring acute inpatient treatment. In these instances, involuntary psychiatric commitment might be the only option available to the emergency physician in providing appropriate care to the patient. Legal precedent in the United States has established a "degree of immediate dangerousness to self or others" threshold as a minimum for involuntary commitment.[1]

The emergency physician should recognize that "commitment involves an infringement of civil liberties" and as such, "relevant laws, regulations, institutional policies, documentation, and patient rights" must all be considered in arriving at the decision for involuntary commitment.[2] The best course of action is the least restrictive treatment option to meet the patient's treatment and security needs, while limiting infringements on the patient's freedom of choice and mobility. Respecting the patient's right to confidentiality and privacy is critical in the evaluation and determination of disposition.[2]

Many patients presenting to the ED for evaluation of involuntary commitment are in the custody of law enforcement. In general, the characteristics and outcomes of patients brought to the ED by police are poorly understood. Patients with involuntary holds who were brought to the ED are more likely to have a longer ED length of stay and more likely to have a presentation related to violence, although they are not more likely to require restraints while in the ED. Patients with involuntary holds are also at risk for escalating into violent behaviors that put healthcare workers and other in the ED at risk. However, there is a lack of data to support the need for restraints in patients brought to the ED by police, underscoring the need to exhaust attempts at the least restrictive approach to patients with acute psychiatric needs presenting to the ED.

Patients who are intoxicated in the ED usually do not meet criteria for having decision-making capacity and, when sober, are often unable to recall discussions of consent. These patients should not be reflexively placed in involuntary status. A cognitive evaluation and, when needed, legal and ethics consultation can assist in decision-making about commitment status. Although medical etiologies for symptoms are less common, they should be considered in evaluating patients deemed to require involuntary psychiatric admission. Final decisions about whether a patient requires involuntary admission for an acute psychiatric presentation should be deferred until a patient has reached sobriety and has had a completed evaluation for organic etiologies of the presenting symptoms. Then his/her decision-making capacity can be reassessed and the patient can have the opportunity to consent to further treatment if necessary.

Patients with involuntary psychiatric hold status can have a considerable impact on the EMS system. In one large study, patients with involuntary hold status represented 10% of all EMS encounters, and many of these patients had higher overall use of EMS.[3] Finally, patients with psychiatric and mental health symptoms are disproportionally impacted by prolonged ED length of stay,[4,5] and this is particularly the case for patients with involuntary commitment status. For example, in Florida, where statute states that patients requiring involuntary psychiatric evaluation must not wait longer than 12 hours to be transferred from an ED, almost half of patients wait longer than the 12 hours mandated by state law.[6,7] Increased ED lengths of stay for patients with involuntary holds are associated with urine drug testing, blood alcohol concentration testing, barbiturates found on urine drug testing, male gender, and insurance status.[6]

The primary goal for the emergency physician is to act in the best interest of the patient, maintaining patient autonomy and dignity. Because involuntary psychiatric commitment involves limitations on a patient's rights to autonomy and liberty, it should be reserved for those exceptional cases in which a patient poses a clear and imminent danger to self or others and does not have the capacity or ability to consent to voluntary treatment. It should never be used as a tool of coercion, to resolve relationship conflicts, or as a therapy for an underlying disease state, particularly in patients suffering from substance or alcohol use disorders. The emergency physician can use "Zeller's six goals"[8] to assist in the management of patients presenting with acute psychiatric needs:

1. Exclude medical etiologies of symptoms and ensure medical stability.
2. Rapidly stabilize the acute crisis.
3. Avoid coercion.
4. Treat in the least restrictive setting.
5. Form a therapeutic alliance.
6. Formulate an appropriate disposition and aftercare plan.

CASE RESOLUTION

The emergency physician should complete an evaluation of the patient to determine whether he has acute psychiatric need that requires either voluntary or involuntary admission for additional evaluation and treatment by a psychiatric team. This evaluation should exclude any medical etiologies for the patient's symptoms. The determination of disposition requires reassessment when the patient exhibits decision-making capacity and is no longer under the influence of alcohol or drugs.

After an extended conversation with the patient, the emergency physician does not elicit any homicidal or suicidal ideations from the patient. The patient admits making a statement about "ending it all," but he reports that this was made during an argument and while intoxicated. He provides the emergency physician with a detailed description of some of the many reasons in his life he has for living: a stable job, a young child, good friends. The patient's significant other has arrived at the ED and provides additional history that the patient has been making suicidal comments more frequently and when he is not intoxicated. She expresses grave concerns about his safety because of his increasingly frequent comments about suicide. The emergency physician cannot definitively determine that the patient is not a risk to himself. The physician makes a clinical judgment that the patient should have inpatient psychiatric evaluation and is compelled by the concerns of the patient's significant other regarding the patient's safety. The patient is offered and declines voluntary psychiatric evaluation, and involuntary commitment is initiated.

An additional, unique, and important issue related to involuntary commitment is its application in the pediatric population. The discussion of involuntary commitment is beyond the scope of this chapter.

KEY POINTS TO REMEMBER

- Patients presenting to the ED with psychiatric complaints should have an evaluation for alternative etiologies of their symptoms if indicated.
- The least restrictive treatment option should be sought.
- Effort should be made to limit infringements on the patient's freedom of choice and mobility.

References

1. Substance Abuse and Mental Health Services Administration (SAMHSA). Civil commitment and the mental health care continuum: Historical trends and principles for law and practice. 2019. https://www.samhsa.gov/sites/default/files/civil-commitment-continuum-of-care.pdf

2. American College of Emergency Physicians. Civil commitment: Policy statement. April 2017. https://www.acep.org/globalassets/new-pdfs/policy-statements/civil.commitment.pdf

3. Trivedi TK, Glenn M, Hern G, et al. Emergency medical services use among patients receiving involuntary psychiatric holds and the safety of an out-of-hospital screening protocol to "medically clear" psychiatric emergencies in the field, 2011–2016. *Ann Emerg Med.* 2019;73(1):42–51.

4. Pearlmutter MD, Dwyer KH, Burke LG, et al. Analysis of emergency department length of stay for mental health patients at ten Massachusetts emergency departments. *Ann Emerg Med.* 2017;70(2):193–202.

5. Misek RK, DeBarba AE, Brill A. Predictors of psychiatric boarding in the emergency department. *West J Emerg Med.* 2015;16(1):71–75.

6. Brennaman L. Exceeding the legal time limits for involuntary mental health examinations: A study of emergency department delays. *Policy Polit Nurs Pract*. 2015;16(3–4):67–78.
7. Brennaman L, Boursaw B, Christy A, Meize-Growchowski R. Delayed access to involuntary mental health examination. *J Behav Health Serv Res*. 2017;44(4):666–683.
8. Zeller SL. Treatment of psychiatric patients in emergency settings. *Primary Psychiatry*. 2010;17:35–41.

Further Reading

Al-Khafaji A, Loy J, Kelly AM. Characteristics and outcome of patients brought to an emergency department by police under the provisions (Section 10) of the Mental Health Act in Victoria, Australia. *Int J Law Psychiatry*. 2014;37(4):415–419.

Crilly J, Johnston AN, Wallis M, et al. Review article: Clinical characteristics and outcomes of patient presentations to the emergency department via police: A scoping review. *Emerg Med Australas*. 2019;31(4):506–515.

Dawson NL, Lachner C, Vadenoncoceur TF, et al. Violent behavior by emergency department patients with an involuntary hold status. *Am J Emerg Med*. 2018;36(3):392–395.

Hedman LC, Petrila J, Fisher WH, et al. State laws on emergency holds for mental health stabilization. *Psychiatr Serv*. 2016;67(5):529–535.

Llewellin P, Arendts, Weeden J, Pethebridge A. Involuntary psychiatric attendances at an Australasian emergency department: A comparison of police and health-care worked initiated presentations. *Emerg Med Australas*. 2011;23(5):593–599.

Maniaci MJ, Lachner C, Vadeboncoeur TF, et al. Involuntary patient length-of-stay at a suburban emergency department. *Am J Emerg Med*. 2020;38(3):534–538.

Martel ML, Klein LR, Miner JR, et al. A brief assessment of capacity to consent instrument in acutely intoxicated emergency department patients. *Am J Emerg Med*. 2018;36(1):18–23.

Miller D. Is involuntary hold for psychiatric patients the only answer? *ACEPNow*, July 10, 2017. https://www.acepnow.com/article/involuntary-hold-psychiatric-patients-answer/

Nassif WM. Assessing decisional capacity in patients with substance use disorders. *Curr Psychiatry*. 2019;18(10):35–40.

Roy A, Lachner C, Dumitrascu A, et al. Patients on involuntary hold status in the emergency department. *South Med J*. 2019;112(5):265–270.

Soliman AE, Reza H. Risk factors and correlates of violence among acutely ill adult psychiatric inpatients. *Psychiatr Serv*. 2001;52(1):75–80.

Substance Abuse and Mental Health Services Administration (SAMHSA). National guidelines for behavioral health crisis care: Best practice toolkit. 2020. https://www.samhsa.gov/sites/default/files/national-guidelines-for-behavioral-health-crisis-care-02242020.pdf

World Health Organization (WHO). Mental health care law: Ten basic principles. 1996. https://www.who.int/mental_health/media/en/75.pdf?ua=1

26 Sick from Waiting

Chadd K. Kraus

A 38-year-old female presents to the ED with
acute suicidal thoughts, without a specific plan.
The patient has a remote history of a suicide
attempt by medication overdose but no evidence
to suggest current suicide attempt or self-injury.
The patient has a documented, longstanding
history of depression and anxiety and is on
several outpatient medications related to these
conditions. She reports several recent life
stressors, including the death of her father and
loss of her job as particularly distressing to her.
After performing a thorough history and physical
exam, the emergency physician determines
that the patient does not have an acute medical
etiology to explain her symptoms and concludes
that the patient would benefit from inpatient
hospitalization for psychiatric evaluation and
treatment.

What do you do now?

BOARDING OF PATIENTS WITH PSYCHIATRIC NEEDS IN THE ED: THE WAIT

Over the past approximately 40 to 50 years, changes in the delivery of psychiatric care in the United States, including a shift to community-based, outpatient care and fewer hospital beds dedicated to psychiatric conditions, have contributed to an increase in acute and general psychiatric and behavioral healthcare provided in EDs. Along with the increase in demand psychiatric care and a relative paucity of psychiatrists and other mental health professionals, EDs have become the safety net for patients with acute psychiatric symptoms and also for patients with complex and chronic psychiatric care needs.

This situation has placed strain on EDs, where patients with acute symptoms of psychiatric illness are frequently "boarded" awaiting inpatient hospitalization for additional care. No single definition exists for boarding, but the term broadly applies to patients in the ED in whom the decision for hospitalization has been made but for whom an inpatient bed in the hospital is not yet available. Boarding in the ED is common for patients with a range of medical and surgical conditions and has been associated with increased patient morbidity and mortality. There are a variety of factors contributing to boarding for patients with psychiatric needs in the ED. System-level challenges (e.g., inpatient bed shortages, lack of community-based resources and alternatives to hospitalization) and patient-level characteristics (e.g., insurance status, housing instability, lack of social support) can all contribute to the pressures on EDs providing acute psychiatric care. Boarding can be particularly detrimental to patients with acute psychiatric presentations. Patients with psychiatric symptoms who are boarded in in the ED are "at an increased risk for symptom exacerbation or elopement."[1] ED patients requiring inpatient psychiatric care have nearly five times higher odds of boarding than patients with non-psychiatric symptoms and are boarded in the ED for almost 3 hours longer.[2] Boarding among pediatric patients awaiting inpatient psychiatric care tends to be even longer than for adults.[3,4] A survey of ED directors showed that nearly 80% of U.S. EDs board patients with psychiatric needs.[5]

For many EDs, providing appropriate and adequate care for these patients can be challenging, particularly in lower-resource hospitals. The majority of U.S. EDs do not have formal psychiatric care or consultations available in the ED. Multiple innovative solutions have been evaluated to reduce psychiatric boarding, including telepsychiatry, psychiatric observation units within an ED, protocols for safe discharge from the ED with rapid outpatient follow-up, patient navigation and case management services, involvement of EMS and mobile crisis units, regional and state registries and tracking systems of available hospital beds, and transfer to regional psychiatric emergency centers. However, such solutions are not feasible in many EDs, particularly those in smaller community hospitals and rural settings, and others require system-level interventions and initiatives that can be resource intensive. Additionally, current reimbursement models present barriers for patients accessing inpatient psychiatric care.

For patients who are boarded in the ED, all possible efforts should be made to expedite disposition. If a patient requires hospitalization and bed availability is delayed, the patient should receive treatment to stabilize their condition within the capabilities of an individual ED. This might include medication initiation or adjustment and should include provision of a patient's home medications. Additionally, the patient should be monitored in the same way as other patients requiring acute, emergency care. Each physician assuming care should document a note regarding the patient's course in the ED. Finally, safe alternatives to hospitalization should be explored.

CASE RESOLUTION

After completing a comprehensive bed search, there is no appropriate inpatient psychiatric bed available for the patient. Because it is late in the evening, the emergency physician discusses with the patient that it could be well into the next day, if not longer, before a bed becomes available. The patient states that she does not want to wait in the ED for that long to have inpatient treatment and thinks she is stable enough to follow up as an outpatient, with an interim adjustment of her outpatient medications as an alternative to inpatient hospitalization.

The emergency physician consults, via phone, the hospital's on-call psychiatrist. They discuss the patient's outpatient medication regimen, presenting symptoms, and current clinical condition in the ED. The psychiatrist recommends medication and dosage adjustments that might benefit the patient in the acute setting. These medications are available and can be administered in the ED.

In determining the patient's disposition, patient autonomy should be respected, and shared decision-making should be employed. All possible efforts should be made to expedite disposition from the ED using the least restrictive available alternative in the patient's best interest. Through a shared decision-making discussion with the patient, she decides that she does not want to remain boarded in the ED awaiting hospitalization. She says her symptoms are improved, and she has good social support and will return to the ED if she worsens. The patient's sister is contacted and arrives at the ED to pick up the patient and assures the emergency physician that she will be staying with the patient for the next few days. Arrangements are made with psychiatry for outpatient follow-up within the next 48 hours. The patient is discharged home in the care of her sister, and with strict return precautions if her symptoms are worsening or new symptoms develop.

KEY POINTS TO REMEMBER

- Boarding of patients with psychiatric needs in the ED is common.
- Patients should be reassessed frequently during their ED stay, and care provided to the patient should be provided at the level of capability of the ED.
- All possible efforts should be made to expedite disposition from the ED using the least restrictive available alternative in the patient's best interest.

References

1. Nicks BA, Manthey DM. The impact of psychiatric boarding in emergency departments. *Emerg Med Int*. 2012;2012:360308.
2. Nolan JM, Fee C, Cooper BA, et al. Psychiatric boarding incidence, duration, and associated factors in United States emergency departments. *J Emerg Nurs*. 2015;41(1):57–64.

3. Yoon J, Bui LN, Govier DJ, et al. Determinants of boarding of patients with severe mental illness in hospital emergency departments. *J Ment Health Policy Econ.* 2020;23(2):61–75

4. McEnany FB, Ojugbele O, Doherty JR, et al. Pediatric mental health boarding. *Pediatrics.* 2020;146(4):e20201174.

5. American College of Emergency Physicians (ACEP). Practical solutions to boarding of psychiatric patients in the emergency department: Does your emergency department have a psychiatric boarding problem? October 2015. https://www.macep.org/Files/Behavioral%20Health%20Boarding/Practical%20Solutions%20to%20Boarding%20of%20Psych%20Patients%20in%20EDs.pdf

Further Reading

Misek RK, DeBarba AE, Brill A. Predictors of psychiatric boarding in the emergency department. *West J Emerg Med.* 2015;16(1):71–75.

Nordstrom K, Berlin JS, Nash SS, et al. Boarding of mentally ill patients in the emergency department: American Psychiatric Association resource document. *West J Emerg Med.* 2019;20(5):690–695.

Parwani V, Tinloy B, Ulrich A, et al. Opening of psychiatric observation unit eases boarding crisis. *Acad Emerg Med.* 2018;25:456–460.

Pearlmutter MD, Dwyer KH, Burke LG, et al. Analysis of emergency department length of stay for mental health patients at ten Massachusetts emergency departments. *Ann Emerg Med.* 2017;70(2):193–202.

Zeller S, Calma N, Stone A. Effects of a dedicated regional psychiatric emergency service on boarding of psychiatric patients in area emergency departments. *West J Emerg Med.* 2014;15(1):1–6.

27 Down with Disease

William A. Johnjulio and Moira Davenport

A 32-year-old male presents to the ED with worsening of his depression, difficulty sleeping, decreased appetite, and suicidal thoughts. The patient had never attempted suicide in the past, but he is now considering jumping off a bridge. The patient has a history of depression and obesity, with no other medical history. He has seen psychologists and psychiatrists in the past but has been having acutely worsening symptoms over the past 3 days. He was unable to schedule an appointment with his psychiatrist. He denies visual hallucinations, but he does have auditory hallucinations with voices that tell him to hurt himself. He is taking sertraline as prescribed. The patient smokes half-a-pack of cigarettes per day but denies alcohol use or illicit drug use. He denies constitutional symptoms, chest pain, shortness of breath, abdominal pain, and urinary or bowel symptoms. There is no reported physical trauma. He denies any focal weakness or paresthesias. Vital signs are HR 80, BP 130/70, RR 14, temp 37°C, SpO_2 99% on room air. Physical examination is normal with the exception of obesity.

What do you do now?

ACCESS TO MENTAL HEALTH CARE

Access to mental health care is a nationwide problem that has a large impact on EDs. Caring for psychiatric patients in the ED is multifaceted. First, the utmost attention must be directed toward assessing for potential medical etiologies that may be causing or contributing to the patient's presentation. Second, consultation with psychiatric specialists is frequently required. Third, an emergency physician must coordinate inpatient and outpatient planning for the patient. Emergency physicians are extremely qualified and adept at assessing for and evaluating medical problems, but they are not trained in the specific intricacies of psychiatric care, such as selecting appropriate long-term medications and the details of appropriate follow-up. Also, inpatient and outpatient resources are highly varied by location, healthcare system, and a patient's insurance status. Combined with emergency physicians being required to simultaneously care for a large volume of patients at once, this highlights the importance of obtaining help from other facets of the healthcare system in caring for psychiatric patients who present to the ED.

The first priority of an emergency physician in evaluating nearly every patient is assessing for critical medical problems that require immediate attention. This begins with assessing the ABCs (airway, breathing, and circulation). Next, a focused history and physical exam is performed. Finally, the physician generates an overall impression and plan for each patient. For psychiatric patients in particular, a careful assessment must be conducted for infectious, metabolic, or any other underlying cause for a patient's presentation. Many potential medical problems can be ruled out with a proper history and physical exam. Emergency physicians are very qualified to make the decision regarding who needs labs and imaging based on the patient's history and physical examination. Many patients, particularly those with a known psychiatric diagnosis and no history of trauma, do not require any labs or imaging. The more difficult aspects of caring for psychiatric patients in the ED are obtaining psychiatric consultation and providing inpatient and outpatient recommendations and treatment. As displayed in the case in this chapter, the patient is experiencing threatening thoughts regarding jumping off a bridge to commit suicide. Determining whether or not this patient is safe for discharge is a complex and high-risk decision faced by the emergency physician. This is a scenario where having help from supporting staff is invaluable.

Many EDs are beginning to see the value in having on-call psychiatry staff, which leads to more rapid evaluation and disposition planning for psychiatric patients. The University of North Carolina created a "Division of Psychiatry" within their ED, using its own psychiatrists, psychiatry social workers, and nurse practitioners. Their protocol is for patients to be seen in the ED within 2 hours. Having these systems in place greatly reduces the time that psychiatric patients are required to spend in the ED, particularly those who are quickly seen by the psychiatry team and then deemed safe for discharge.

Other national emergency medicine provider groups are vetting processes to provide telemedicine platforms to care for psychiatric patients in the ED. Telemedicine psychiatrists can help evaluate and provide disposition guidance for many patients. Many psychiatric patients are required to board in EDs until business hours, when the psychiatry team is available for consult. Having telemedicine psychiatrists reduces the number of patients who are required to board in the ED during non-business hours. Telemedicine and in-house staff can also help emergency physicians initiate early medication therapy for psychiatric patients who experience long boarding times while awaiting inpatient placement. Providing 24-hour psychiatric coverage through in-house staff or with telemedicine capabilities is an excellent method for EDs and for healthcare systems as a whole to improve access to mental health care.

Involving social workers and case managers in the care of psychiatric patients can be paramount to obtaining the appropriate follow-up for these patients. Cohen and colleagues showed that 38% of Americans had to wait over 1 week to get mental health treatment and 46% had to travel over 1 hour round trip to get to an appointment. Additionally, 46% of those who didn't seek treatment cited that not knowing where to seek treatment was the main deterrent against seeking help.[1] This puts a lot of people at risk of using the ED for their psychiatric care. Specifically, homeless populations and people without insurance are, on average, higher utilizers of EDs and have their own unique barriers to obtaining mental health care. Estimates show that 30% of homeless populations have some type of mental illness, and around 70% have at least mild cognitive impairement.[2,3] These patient populations also have higher rates of certain medical diseases, including skin and dental infections, respiratory disease, sexually transmitted infections (STIs), and illicit drug addiction, to name a few. Emergency physicians must maintain a high level of suspicion that underlying pathology may be contributing to the patient's acute or worsening psychiatric presentation. This also presents a unique challenge for coordinating outpatient follow-up. Social workers and case managers are able to help patients navigate varying insurance coverages and provide a list of outpatient medical and housing resources in the surrounding area. Engaging these hospital personnel is a crucial aspect in allowing the emergency physician to focus on high volumes and critical patients that make up the rest of their department.

Many hospitals also have separate holding areas for psychiatric patients in the ED. A separate psychiatric holding area is beneficial, as it can be staffed by those who are specially trained to manage psychiatric patients. This is an important concept, as psychiatric patients are four to six times more likely to have out-of-network coverage compared to medical or surgical patients and thus often require transfer to another facility, prolonging boarding times for psychiatric patients awaiting inpatient placement. These separate areas also keep psychiatric patients away from the main ED area, which is often loud and contains bright lights and frequent activity, all of which can be disturbing and a trigger to worsen a patient's presenting condition. Patients should be screened for weapons and other contraband in these areas (as well as in the general ED), preferably by specialty staff who are sensitive to many unique needs of psychiatric patients.

Another area where telemedicine and mobile apps may hold potential for future improvement involves outpatient planning. A systematic literature review analyzed 4,658 patients who were engaged in their healthcare by SMS text or mobile apps. Intervention was provided for anxiety, depression, stress, weight management, and smoking cessation during pregnancy. This study showed promising efficacy for mobile interventions.[4] Another study followed pediatric patients, age 7 to 19, who were seen by a psychiatry consult team in the ED. The study found that only 73% of these pediatric patients were able to establish outpatient psychiatric care within 1 month.[5] This is another area where having a healthcare system that uses SMS text or mobile apps to engage patients in follow-up care may improve patients' access to mental health care.

Overall, patients who present to the ED with psychiatric complaints are a unique population and require a specific set of skills and resources. Again, the importance of adequate medical clearance cannot be overemphasized. The emergency physician must obtain a focused history and physical exam and keep a wide differential of potential causes for the patient's presentation. Once medical etiologies are ruled out, with or without further testing, the next step is often dependent upon psychiatric consultation. This is frequently required to determine if a patient is safe for discharge. In-house psychiatrists who are available for consult are invaluable. Telemedicine also has a strong potential to be used in this area of emergency medicine. Creating a dedicated psychiatric part of the ED with a specialized set of staff and environment is another potential area to improve patient experience. Having social workers and case managers assist in outpatient planning is essential, and understanding your community resources will prove to be beneficial as well. Telemedicine techniques such as SMS texting or mobile apps are potential areas for our psychiatrist colleagues to improve their outpatient follow-up, as studies have demonstrated promising efficacy.

Ultimately, each psychiatric case will have its unique challenges; the emergency physician should learn from each case. We encourage readers to engage their emergency medicine colleagues and hospital administration to improve the systems that are in place to care for psychiatric patients who present to the ED. We have noted potential ways to improve patients' access to mental health care.

CASE RESOLUTION

The patient was first seen and evaluated by an emergency physician, who, through history and physical examination, cleared the patient for psychiatric evaluation and disposition. Fortunately, this patient was seen in an ED that has access to 24-hour psychiatry consultation. This occurs in person or through telemedicine. The patient was assessed by a psychiatry nurse and psychiatry attending physician. The psychiatry team determined that the patient did not require admission for his current suicidal thoughts and plan. They provided patient counseling in the ED. They also provided the patient with outpatient resources and follow-up appointments. The patient was agreeable with this plan and was discharged from the ED.

- As an emergency physician, you are not alone in being frustrated with the lack of mental health care resources. ED throughput is being interrupted nationwide due to this crisis.
- Work with your ED directors and hospital administration to put systems and operations in place to improve the care provided to psychiatric patients in your ED.
- One of the most important actions is to increase your on-call psychiatry team. This can be through telecommunication or in-person staff. They provide the most help in disposition planning for patients. They can help with determining who is safe for discharge and can help with medication administration for boarders awaiting inpatient beds.
- Know your local outpatient resources that provide psychiatric crisis aid and know the shelters for homeless populations. The majority of patients will not require hospital admission, so outpatient resources are key.

Further Reading

Bagget TP, Kertesz SG, Schwenk TL, Kunins L. Health care of people experiencing homelessness in the United States. UpToDate. June 19, 2020. https://www.uptodate.com/contents/health-care-of-people-experiencing-homelessness-in-the-united-states?search=homelessness%20and%20mental%20illness&sectionRank=2&usage_type=default&anchor=H12138178&source=machineLearning&selectedTitle=1~150&display_rank=1#H12138154

Cohen Veterans Network and National Council for Behavioral Health. America's Mental Health 2018. October 2018. https://www.cohenveteransnetwork.org/wp-content/uploads/2018/10/Research-Summary-10-10-2018.pdf

Kalter L. Treating mental illness in the ED. AAMC. September 3, 2019. https://www.aamc.org/news-insights/treating-mental-illness-ed

Murrell K, Klauer K, Horst J, Powell E. Beyond boarding: A new paradigm for mental health care in the emergency department. TEAMHealth white paper. May 2019. https://www.teamhealth.com/wp-content/uploads/2019/05/TH-11829-White-Paper_BHinED_20190426.pdf

Rathbone AL, Prescott J. The use of mobile apps and SMS messaging as physical and mental health interventions: Systematic review. *J Med Internet Res.* 2017;19(8):e295. doi:10.2196/jmir.7740

28 I Would Like to Phone a Friend

David Hoke and Bryan Balentine

This evening, you are working in a rural critical access ED. A 31-year-old male with a history of depression and anxiety presents tonight with his roommate for a complaint of worsening sadness. His roommate reports that, this afternoon, the patient expressed a desire to overdose on drugs. Of note, the patient does not have a significant drug history nor ready access to drugs. The patient reports he broke up with a girlfriend and was very upset this afternoon. He acknowledged what he said, and that he did feel that way at the time, but that he does not want to hurt himself now. He does feel that he is still more sad than normal. He takes Lexapro (escitalopram) 10 mg daily and has been taking it as normal. He does not have any guns. He has an outpatient psychiatrist who only sees patients in town once a week and will not be available for several days. There is no on-call psychiatrist for your hospital. The closest psychiatric facility is a 3-hour drive away.

What do you do now?

TELEPSYCHIATRY

You call the telepsychiatrist, for whom you prudently advocated over the last year. This case highlights a patient who has demonstrated true and concerning symptoms, recently, in regard to depression. You are thankful that his roommate encouraged him to seek help at your ED, as the patient certainly required evaluation. However, the patient has now improved somewhat from his earlier status, and you deem him not to be a risk to himself or anyone else at this moment. He seems reasonable and goal-oriented, with good insight. He does not have many specific risk factors in terms of access to agents of overdose or firearms. However, he does have significant stressors in his life that are triggers for his earlier concerning statements. At this time, with support of his roommate and with the guidance or your medical staff, he is not intending, nor expressing, a desire to hurt himself. You are rightly, however, concerned about his course over the next few days, without continued support and further evaluation, including possible medication changes. While appreciative of the roommate, you do not feel that you can count on this person to provide all necessary support, and the patient reports few friends and no family in the area. Since the patient is not a risk to himself, you do not feel that commitment is necessary, nor would a voluntary admission for emergent psychiatric evaluation truly be warranted at this juncture. However, you do feel that urgent, rather than emergent, evaluation is necessary. Unfortunately, this is unlikely to occur after discharge in the outpatient setting, given your rural location and infrequent visits by the patient's psychiatrist. Like so many small hospitals in America, you lack in-person psychiatric resources at your hospital.

Such a situation is a perfect opportunity to use telepsychiatry. Telepsychiatry falls under the larger umbrella of telemedicine and, further, telehealth. Telehealth is a growing mode of delivery for a variety of medical fields. The American Telemedicine Association describes telehealth as technology-enabled health and care management and delivery systems that extend capacity and access. Telehealth can take many forms and in general refers to any remote transmittance of health information from one site to another. It can be in the form of videoconference, asynchronous transmittal (such as radiology studies sent to be read at a later time), or remote patient monitoring (such as intensivist monitoring of vital signs in an ICU, with no attending physician present overnight).

Telepsychiatry, more specifically, can also take many forms. It often involves videoconferencing, usually between a psychiatrist or other mental health professional and a patient. This can be for a scheduled appointment that patients can make on their own, in an inpatient setting to support psychiatric evaluation of general medical admissions at sites without psychiatrists, or in the ED. There are even programs that allow schoolchildren to have specialist appointments from their schools, conferencing with the doctor at their office, and with their parents from work. Through these videoconferenced interviews, psychiatrists can provide essentially all of the same services from a remote location that they would otherwise be able to provide in person. They can evaluate the patient to support your decision for a safe discharge or recommend admission and transfer. They can make medication recommendations and many times actually prescribe the medications themselves, since they must be licensed in the state in which the patient is being seen. Moreover, they can arrange further disposition or follow-up, sometimes coordinating admission to their own inpatient facilities, or outpatient follow-up through their own office, a known local colleague, or another at-home videoconference.

The benefits here are obvious. According to the American Psychiatric Association:

> Telepsychiatry is helping bring more timely psychiatric care to emergency departments. An estimated one in eight emergency department visits involves a mental health and/or substance use condition, according to the Agency for Healthcare Research and Quality. Many emergency departments are not equipped to handle people with serious mental health issues and do not have psychiatrists or other mental health clinicians on staff to assess and treat mental health problems. A 2016 poll of emergency physicians found only 17 percent reported having a psychiatrist on call to respond to psychiatric emergencies.[1]

Moreover, emergency physicians in one study reported inability or lack of resources available to treat mental health emergencies in terms of evaluation, proper disposition, and treatment without available mental health–specific resources.[2] Lastly, this is a growing problem, as psychiatric presentations represent the fastest-growing component of emergency medicine patients.

Evidence supports ED utilization of telepsychiatry. The technology has come to the point where its use is quite feasible. Limitations such as patients' hearing, concentration, or attention are easily overcome. Most areas have appropriate connectivity; however, some rural areas may still require patients to travel to receive a better connection, though this may be far closer than traveling to see the mental health professional. Moreover, its use has been validated: "Diagnoses have been made reliably, with good inter-rater reliability, for a wide range of psychiatric disorders in children, adolescents, and adults; less information is available on geriatric patients, but preliminary results are positive."[3] There are some limitations in certain patient populations, such as the severely autistic and the elderly who may be resistant to use of the technology. Other patient populations, such as adolescents, have been found to respond better, possibly due to the novel use of technology and their comfort with it.

Telemedicine use is effective, especially in the ED. In a review of five sites, it was found that most consultations occurred when the request was made, and nearly all within 1 hour, each lasting 5 to 10 minutes. The most common diagnoses evaluated were major depression, bipolar disorder, and schizophrenia or schizoaffective disorder. All programs either discharged patients with scheduled follow-up, admitted them, or transferred the patients to a specialty facility. A University of Mississippi program provided details that are potentially practice-changing for many EDs that experience long transfer times just for evaluation: 65% were discharged, 16% were admitted, and 19% were transferred.[4]

Use of telepsychiatry improves ease of disposition and facilitates ED flow. One study of a statewide implementation system for telepsychiatry in South Carolina showed a markedly decreased length of stay for psychiatric patients, from 1.35 to 0.43 days.[5] As many small EDs may have 15 beds or less, this increases ED bed availability and frees staff resources from a single patient who, by sitting in the ED, is getting minimal treatment. Combined with the additional costs required by such patients, often including one-to-one observation, the cost savings is huge. This may, in turn, lead to an increase in bed turnover, better patient throughput, and a decrease in patients who leave without being seen. In the same study, these patients were found to have 30-day-follow-up rates of 46% versus only 16% in matched groups. Additionally, a drop in admissions of 22% to 11% was shown for those assessed by telepsychiatry. Lower inpatient costs and overall 30-day health-care costs were also demonstrated.[5]

Establishing a telepsychiatry program is relatively easy in comparison to starting brick-and-mortar practices. Psychiatrists must be licensed in the state in which the patient is seen. While the psychiatrist must be credentialed at each hospital, a streamlined credentialing process can be used if hospitals have credentialing agreements that allow a second hospital to accept the full credential process of a primary facility. As with standard visits, two bills will be generated: both a facility fee and a professional fee. How the physician is reimbursed can vary. The facility may do all of the billing and contract with a provider or group and pay them a flat rate per encounter or a monthly fee based on average volume. Facility-employed psychiatrists may simply assume this as part of their duties. Lastly, psychiatrists may bill their own professional fees directly from the payer.

Reimbursement policies are generally driven by state regulations, so feasibility will need to be assessed on a local level. Whether using public or private insurance, many states have geographic limitations for telehealth. These can include critical access hospital designations, physical distance between patient and professional, or specified low-resource areas. Generally, Medicaid allows for state implementation and interpretation, although 48 states allow for reimbursement of some telepsychiatry services. For Medicare, standard members are covered for videoconferencing in rural areas. Many Medicare managed plans have broader access. Private payers are subject both to state regulations and their own interpretation. Twenty-four states have parity laws for telemedicine services. Sixteen states have full coverage and have no restrictions based upon professionals' geographic location or type of technology. Increasingly, managed care organizations are partnering with organizations that can provide 24/7 coverage for specialty services such as telepsychiatry. Pandemic outbreaks have prompted the relaxation of regulations regarding reimbursement of videoconferencing temporarily, and it will be interesting to observe the evolution of telemedicine and permanent changes to policy, given major disturbances in health and healthcare, of this sort.

Several technological considerations must be addressed to employ this service; however, they are generally met without much challenge at this point in technical evolution. Upload and download speeds of at least 5 mbps are required to avoid pixilation and interruptions. Requirements may be higher depending upon the system deployed. The platform must be HIPAA complaint. Physicians cannot use standard FaceTime, Skype, or Google Meet applications available to the general public, as these are not considered secure. To meet HIPAA compliance, the platform must meet the following criteria: encryption meeting FIPS 140-2 certified 256 bit standard; peer-to-peer videoconferencing is not stored or intercepted by the company; and any storage that may be performed is done locally on a HIPAA-compliant device. (These restrictions may also change following COVID-related policy changes.) Services and platforms can vary widely. Some platforms advertise full practice support for the psychiatrist with EMR, billing, and even scribing. One company advertises platforms that use existing hardware such as home computers or tablets for secure chats. Others sell carts with considerable capability, including physician control of camera and even auscultation technologies. This may be more hardware than necessary to start up a telepsychiatry service but would allow multiple uses such as teleneurology, telecardiology, telepulmonology, and teleintensive care.

Practice models vary widely. A single psychiatrist or group can contract services on their own with a facility, or partner with a third-party vendor to provide the logistics for their service. Having a local group provide the service can be beneficial, as they will often cover several facilities nearby, will know the local healthcare system well, and can more easily establish follow-up, whether transfer, admission (often to their own facilities where they will see the patient), or outpatient follow-up that will accept the patient's insurance (whether public option or sometimes in their own office). However, a small local group can be less stable, or less able to provide 24/7 coverage. Larger telepsychiatry groups generally have a more streamlined process and a larger number of psychiatrists who can easily be available, but they may not be as aware of local resources. Lastly, some large systems may employ a spoke-and-wheel model where the larger tertiary facilities provide coverage to smaller outlying facilities and have the advantage of close working relationships and maintaining patients within the system.[4]

Telepsychiatry is a useful tool for resource-poor areas. It provides faster evaluation and treatment for mental health emergencies; it decreases patient length of stay, healthcare costs, and ED burden overall. It is relatively easy to employ and requires only moderate technological considerations that may already be present at your institution. The time to advocate for its use is now, before you have the patient in front of you.

CASE RESOLUTION

The patient was interviewed by the psychiatrist over the telecart. The patient maintained that he no longer wished to hurt himself. The psychiatrist recommended increasing the dose of escitalopram to 20 mg daily and sent the prescription electronically to the patient's pharmacy. The psychiatrist, who is part of a large local group, was able to organize a follow-up phone appointment with a therapist the next day and scheduled a follow-up appointment with the patient's psychiatrist during her next local session. The patient contracted for safety and his roommate agreed to stay home with him until the follow-up call tomorrow.

KEY POINTS TO REMEMBER

- Psychiatric crisis patients are high-risk dispositions.
- Consultation with a psychiatrist supports your disposition and can help ensure safe discharge and ensure follow-up.
- In resource-limited areas, advocating for a telepsychiatric service can provide psychiatric services where they would have otherwise never existed and can limit unnecessary long transfers and admission.

References

1. American Psychiatric Association. What is telepsychiatry? January 2017. https://www.psychiatry.org/patients-families/what-is-telepsychiatry

2. Meyer JD, McKean AJS, Blegen RN, Demaerschalk BM. Emergency department telepsychiatry service model for a rural regional health system: The first steps. *Telemed J E Health*. 2019;25(1):18–24.

3. Hilty DM, Ferrer DC, Parish MB, et al. The effectiveness of telemental health: A 2013 review. *Telemed J E Health*. 2013;19(6):444–454.

4. Williams M, Pfeffer M, Boyle J, Hilty DM. Telepsychiatry in the emergency department. California Health Care

Foundation. December 2009. https://www.chcf.org/publication/
telepsychiatry-in-the-emergency-department-overview-and-case-studies/

5. Narasimhan M, Druss BG, Hockenberry JM, et al. Impact of a telepsychiatry
program at emergency departments statewide on the quality, utilization, and
costs of mental health services. *Psychiatr Serv.* 2015;66(11):1167–1172.

Further Reading

American Telemedicine Association. Telehealth basics. https://www.americantelemed.
org/resource/why-telemedicine/

American Psychiatric Association. Telepsychiatry toolkit. https://www.psychiatry.org/
psychiatrists/practice/telepsychiatry/toolkit

Updox. HIPAA-compliant video chat. https://www.updox.com/solutions/telehealth/
video-chat/

29 Right into the Danger Zone

Arthur R. Derse

A man who appears to be in his 30s is brought in by EMS from a bus station because of agitation, talking to himself and saying that "there are those who should be very afraid of me." When he is brought to the ED, he is awake and alert, his vital signs are normal, and he says he has no pain or discomfort. He is oriented to person, place, and time. He allows his blood to be drawn. There are no past records available. He denies any suicidal ideation, but when asked if he might harm others, he says, "There are those who should be very afraid of me. They testified against me and I was locked up. If I have the opportunity, I will kill them." When asked who and under what circumstances, he refuses to go into any more detail. His physical exam is unremarkable. His initial labs show no alcohol or drugs. He wants to leave.

What do you do now?

ETHICAL ISSUES IN EMERGENCY PSYCHIATRY

Consent for Treatment and Informed Consent

For over a century, since the *Schloendorff* case,[1] consent has been required for a clinician to provide treatment to a patient. The mere need for treatment does not allow clinicians to treat the patient without his/her consent. The principle was established that "every human being of adult years and sound mind has a right to determine what shall be done" with one's own body. Unconsented treatment might be cause for charges of battery. The *Salgo* case,[2] decided over 50 years ago, requires that offered treatment should come with a description of the nature of the procedure, the risks of the treatment both common and severe, alternative treatments available, and the effect of choosing to forgo treatment. In the case here, the initial cooperation to be seen by the emergency physician implies consent for evaluation. However, the patient's informed consent usually would be necessary for proposed treatment with medication and most other interventions.

Refusal of Treatment

A series of legal cases support the proposition that patients with decision-making capacity may refuse treatment, including life-sustaining medical treatment. Such life-sustaining medical treatment could encompass resuscitation, ventilators, artificial nutrition and hydration, blood products, and others.

Psychiatric Consent and Forced Treatment

Despite the precedent of consent being required for treatment, in the past, patients who were determined to have psychiatric diseases were routinely subjected to forced treatment without permission based on the proposition that the disease interfered with their ability to understand the need for treatment. In the 1960s, patients began winning the legal right to refuse psychiatric treatment unless they were determined to be an imminent danger to themselves or others. This freed vast numbers of patients who had been confined and treated, and some of these patients were able to be successfully treated as outpatients. However, many individuals with some forms of mental illness found themselves lacking shelter and sustenance while still suffering from their underlying mental diseases.

Nonetheless, patients' right to refuse medical treatment now includes their right to refuse psychiatric treatment, unless they pose an imminent danger to themselves (i.e., a substantial probability of physical harm to self, manifested by evidence of recent threats of or attempts at suicide or serious bodily harm) or an imminent danger to others. "Imminent danger to others" may be defined as a substantial probability of physical harm to other persons as manifested by evidence of recent homicidal or other violent behavior on his/her part, or by evidence that others are placed in reasonable fear of violent behavior and serious physical harm to them, as evidenced by a recent overt act, attempt, or threat to do serious physical harm.

In some states, patients may also be detained if by reason of their mental illness they are unable to satisfy basic needs for nourishment, medical care, shelter, or safety without prompt and adequate treatment so that a substantial probability exists that death, serious physical injury, serious physical debilitation, or serious physical disease will imminently ensue unless the individual receives prompt and adequate treatment for the mental illness.

Competency versus Decisional Capacity

The patient's right to refuse medical treatment is now established for the patient who has the ability to make considered judgments to accept or refuse. Competency determinations are usually judicial determinations of permanent incompetency based on expert psychiatric or mental health testimony. A person is presumed competent until proven otherwise. An adult patient who has been determined to be incompetent in a legal proceeding would then have an appointment of a guardian of the person, a guardian of the estate (including financial matters), or both.

Besides competency determinations, patients may temporarily lack the ability to make medical decisions even if they have not been found to be incompetent by a court. This ability, known as decision-making capacity, is a determination that any clinician should be able to make at a basic level. Decision-making capacity has three basic elements:

1. The ability to comprehend information about the disease, the proposed treatment, and its alternatives, including no treatment
2. The ability to weigh the choices against the patient's values, to appreciate the consequence, and to make an autonomous and

reasoned determination (i.e., an autonomous choice among these alternatives). The choice should be consistent over time, taking into account that patients may change their minds, but the choice shouldn't be random.

3. The ability to communicate a choice to the treatment team.

An analogy that is often used is that of a computer with the ability to take in information, weigh it against an internal set of values, arrive at an outcome, and communicate that outcome. Of course, human beings are not computers, and they make decisions dependent upon their personal beliefs, philosophy, and religious view. The decisions are often made in the context of family, community, and society. Their values may change over time.

Critics often point out that clinicians only are concerned with evaluating decision-making capacity when patients go against their medical advice. This is often true because clinicians presume the ability to make decisions, and when a patient decides to go against medical advice and there are serious and even dire consequences, the clinician understandably should want to ensure that the patient has the ability to make that decision. A determination of decision-making capacity should be evaluated in each clinical encounter. In the given case, the clinician should make a formal evaluation of the patient's ability to make medical decisions, including the ability to refuse treatment.

Confidentiality

The duty of confidentiality for physicians is one that is millennia old, reaching back to a Hippocratic proscription against speaking of information publicly that should be held as confidential. This duty of confidentiality has also been upheld in state statutes and legal decisions. HIPAA has enforced privacy regulations at a federal level to prevent clinicians and other so-called covered entities from disclosing protected health information inappropriately about the patient.

However, public health laws and regulations recognized that there are exceptions to confidentiality warranted for reasons to protect others, such as to prevent the transmission of infectious disease. For instance, a patient with tuberculosis who wished to keep the disease confidential would learn from the physician that public health officials must be informed of the patient's disease in order to prevent transmission to others. The ethical rationale was that physicians owe a duty to others in the community to prevent foreseeable harm to them.

Breach of Confidentiality and Duty to Protect/Warn

The principle of duty to the community was extended into the mental health realm in the landmark case of *Tarasoff* (Calif. 1976), in which clinicians were held to a duty to breach confidentiality when the patient poses significant risk of harm to others. The clinicians had a duty to inform authorities who have public health and safety responsibility. The duty might also extend to a duty to warn an individual whom the clinician learned was at risk of harm from the patient. This California case was adopted by many other states through common law or statute. This placed a new duty of clinicians to assess the likelihood of a patient causing harm to self or others, and based on that determination, to ask for emergency detention of the patient for confinement to prevent harm to others who might be at risk. The duty extended beyond mental health situations. For instance, an emergency physician's evaluation that a school bus driver who was intoxicated and who wanted to leave the ED to drive the school bus that day posed an imminent risk to others might result in a justified breach of confidentiality to prevent the foreseeable harm.

In the case example at the beginning of this chapter, the determination of the likelihood of risk to a potential individual who might be harmed is difficult to assess. The physician should take into account the harm that is posed, who might be harmed, the likelihood of that harm, what the clinician might need to do to attempt to prevent that harm, and the likelihood that the intervention would prevent the harm, and whether the physician should contact authorities, the individual(s) at risk, if known, or both.

Determination of Danger to Self or Others

Risk factors for dangerousness to self include suicidal ideation, prior suicide attempts, family history of suicide, suicide of companions, friends, alcohol and drug abuse, depression, mania, chronic disease and disability, lack of access to behavioral health care, and social isolation. Risk factors for dangerousness to others include an individual history of violence, abuse to self or others, paranoid delusions, hallucinations, and mania, alcohol and drug abuse, lack of access to behavioral health care, and social isolation.

Despite these correlative factors, individual determination of dangerousness to self or others is fraught with uncertainty. Studies have shown that clinicians do not have a high degree of accuracy in prediction. However, there have been many incidents of patients who have caused harm who had been evaluated previously by ED or psychiatric personnel who had determined that the degree of danger did not meet the threshold of detention or reporting during the evaluation. This is a very difficult situation for emergency physicians and mental health professionals who perform emergency evaluations. Nonetheless, emergency physicians must make these determinations as best as possible under the circumstances.

Appropriate security precautions should be in place while taking the history and physical examination. The emergency physician should take care during the evaluation to keep between the patient and a means of exit should the patient become aggressive or combative.

EDs and psychiatric emergency facilities are considered the front line in protecting so-called third parties from dangerous patients as well as protecting dangerous patients from themselves.

Emergency Detention Statutes and Regulations

Many states have applicable statutes that set standards for emergency detention and emergency treatment of patients who pose risks to self or others. In some states, physicians and other clinicians may make a determination that the patient should be detained. In other states, law enforcement personnel must make the determination based on behavior or statements that the officer has witnessed or must be based on an evaluation of a physician or other healthcare personnel. The latter occurs where states have determined that only law enforcement officers should have the police powers of the state to be able to detain a patient involuntarily. In these states, physicians have sometimes been frustrated when the patient has made statements to the physician, but upon interview with the officer the patient denies those statements, or when the officer's determination of the patient's likelihood of dangerousness does not align with that of the physician. The emergency physician is advised to know and understand the applicable state statutes for the practice region.

Involuntary Treatment

Statutes usually specify under what circumstances a patient who is emergently detained may be treated against his/her wishes, and these vary from state to state. The criteria for emergency detention often include that the patient is suffering from a treatable mental disease or defect and poses an imminent threat to self or others. The patient is usually detained for a defined amount of time, and an emergency hearing before a judge will be set to determine whether the patient should continue to be detained for further evaluation and potential treatment. Emergency clinicians and mental health professionals may be asked to testify at such a hearing. In addition, states sometimes also have separate laws that apply to the standards for involuntary treatment of the patients with psychotropic medications. In some states, forcible treatment with psychotropic medications of a patient detained for danger to self or others may be allowed. In other states, patients who are detained emergently for danger to self or others may still have the right to refuse treatment with psychotropic medications, unless there is a judicial order or other authorization.

CASE RESOLUTION

The emergency physician in the case presented has a daunting task of determining (1) the decision-making capacity of the patient to be able to accept or refuse treatment, (2) whether the patient has a psychiatric disorder, and (3) whether the patient is an imminent danger to himself or to others. The clinician will need to ask probing questions about the specifics of the harm that is threatened, the severity of the harm, the likelihood of that harm, and whether there are specific individuals who are threatened. Based on that evaluation, if the patient is an imminent danger to self or others, the clinician must breach confidentiality and contact the appropriate authorities and make an attestation that the patient poses such a danger. If the patient is unwilling to cooperate for a determination of decision-making capacity and risk to self or others, given the patient's threatening statement, restraint of the patient from leaving using the least restrictive means may be appropriate until a determination can be made.

In this case, the emergency physician was unsure of the patient's decision-making capacity, but the patient was cooperative with the physical examination and blood and urine testing. Laboratory examination showed no abnormalities or levels of intoxicants or drugs.

The patient was unwilling to communicate more on the specifics of the threat, though the physician suspected the patient may have an underlying psychiatric disorder. The threat itself was evaluated by the emergency physician as a possibly credible threat of potential imminent danger to unspecified other individuals. On this basis, the emergency physician initiated an involuntary mental health hold for further evaluation of the patient. The emergency physician was prepared to restrain the patient until police came. The patient was not told about the plan until arrival of the police. At this point the patient became extremely combative and was restrained and admitted involuntarily in accord with state law. It was discovered that the patient used a pseudonym when he registered in the ED. Once the patient's identity was determined, medical records from another institution showed an extensive psychiatric history with paranoid ideation, as well as a history of domestic partner abuse and conviction and imprisonment for assault and battery to a neighbor who attempted to intervene in one of the abuse episodes.

The evaluation of patients with potential psychiatric emergencies is fraught with ethical and legal challenges. No clinician has perfect evaluation predictability skills. The physician will be held to the standard of the prudent physician in the same specialty who is similarly situated. If a retrospective review of the adequacy of the provision of the standard of care is undertaken, the documentation in the medical record will help the clinician to explain and defend his/her actions.

KEY POINTS TO REMEMBER

- Patients with decision-making capacity who understand the consequences may refuse evaluation and treatment even for life-threatening conditions.
- Emergency physicians owe patients a duty of confidentiality, but that duty can and should be breached if the patient poses a significant risk of serious harm to self or others.
- Depending upon state statutes or common law, patients who pose a significant risk of harm to self or others may be

emergently detained for treatment of psychiatric illness or for intervention by law enforcement to prevent harm.
- Depending upon state statutes or common law, emergency physicians may have a duty to notify authorities and warn those at risk for harm.

References

1. *Schloendorff v. Society of New York Hospital*, 105 N.E. 92 (N.Y. 1914) at 93, 211 N.Y. 125.
2. *Salgo v. Leland Stanford Jr. Board of Trustees*, 154 Cal.App.2d 560, 317 P.2d 170 (1957).

Further Reading

Battaglia J. Is this patient dangerous? 5 steps to assess risk for violence. *Current Psychiatry*. 2004;3(2):14–21.

Dastidar JG, Odden A. How do I determine if my patient has decision-making capacity? *The Hospitalist*. 2011;2011(8).

National Council of State Legislatures. Mental health professionals' duty to warn. 2018. https://www.ncsl.org/research/health/mental-health-professionals-duty-to-warn.aspx

Substance Abuse and Mental Health Services Administration. Civil commitment and the mental health care continuum: Historical trends and principles for law and practice. 2019. https://www.samhsa.gov/sites/default/files/civil-commitment-continuum-of-care.pdf

Suicide Prevention Resource Center. Risk and protective factors. https://www.sprc.org/about-suicide/risk-protective-factors

Tarasoff v. Regents of University of California, 17 Cal. 3d 425, 551 P.2d 334, 131 Cal. Rptr. 14 (Cal. 1976). https://law.justia.com/cases/california/supreme-court/3d/17/425.html

Treatment Advocacy Center. State standards for civil commitment. Updated September 2020. https://www.treatmentadvocacycenter.org/storage/documents/state-standards/state-standards-for-civil-commitment.pdf

Index

Tables, figures, and boxes are indicated by *t*, *f*, and *b* following the page number

cardiovascular collapse, 68
cardiovascular depression, 21
catecholamine surges, 67
Center for Medicare and Medicaid Services, 116, 151
chemical ingestion behavior, 52
chemical restraint. *See also* antipsychotics; physical (manual) restraint
    common IM medications used for, 27*t*
    factors for consideration, 28
    for pediatric patients, 116
    use for agitated patients, 24–26, 28
citizen-police encounters, 68
Civil Rights Act, Title VI, 167
clonidine, 103
coagulative necrosis, 55
cocaine abuse, 65, 66, 67
cognitive behavioral therapy (CBT)
    for anorexia nervosa, 143
    for borderline personality disorder, 104
    for bulimia nervosa, 134, 135
    for depression, 89
    for schizophrenia, 81
    for self-harm (NSSI), 56
    for somatic symptom disorders, 146, 147
cognitive biases, 31
cognitive disorders/impairment, 37, 108, 110, 118
    differential diagnosis, 127
    laboratory/radiographic evaluation, 127–128
    management, 128–129
    patient history, 124–125
    physical examination, 126–127
cognitive evaluation, 13, 111
cognitive exam/judgment, 6–7*b*, 13, 111
Coin in the Hand Test (CIH test), 159–160
Columbia Protocol, 121
Columbia Suicide Severity Rating Scale (C-SSRS), 38, 39*f*, 40*f*, 41*f*, 121
community-based outpatient care, 182
Community Mental Health Act (1963), 151
computed tomography (CT) studies, 80

confusion
    in elderly adults, 108, 111–113
    possible causes, 108
    in Wernicke's encephalopathy, 153
Confusion Assessment Method (CAM), 111
congestive heart failure exacerbation, 60
counseling
    lethal means counseling, 42–43
    for schizophrenic patients, 81
    for substance use disorders, 77
Cultural Formulation Interview (CFI) section (DSM-5), 166–167
cultural idioms of distress, 167
culturally competent emergency care, 166–171
    assessments, 167
    bridging cultural gaps, 166
    culture shock of patients, 166–167
    ED management, 168–170
    PSYCH mnemonic, 168
culture shock, 166–167
cutting injuries, 52, 53
cystocerebral syndrome, 111

D2 dopamine antagonist, 81–82
de-escalation strategies
    for dangerously violent patients, 116
    hierarchy of needs and, 19–20
    for homicidal patients, 62
    verbal de-escalation, 24, 26, 27, 30
deflection techniques, 119–120, 122
dehydration
    anorexia nervosa and, 140
    bulimia nervosa and, 134
    delirium and, 112
    physical restraining and, 31–32
delirium
    dehydration and, 112
    in elderly adults, 108–113
    environmental factors for, 112
    in excited delirium syndrome, 67–72
    ketamine and, 27*t*
    polypharmacy and, 112
    psychiatric history review for, 4

schizophrenia (*cont.*)
   features/symptoms, 80
   paranoid-type, 17–22
   in pediatric patients, 120
   psychosis and, 29
   schizoid personality disorder, 101
   treatment plan, 81–83
schizotypical personality disorder, 101
scratching behavior, 52
seizures
   in autism spectrum disorders, 125
   in bipolar disorder, 92
   in conversion disorder, 160
   in elderly people, 108
   in homicidal patients, 60
   in schizophrenic patients, 80
selective serotonin reuptake inhibitors
   (SSRIs)
   for anorexia nervosa, 143
   for bulimia nervosa, 134–136
   for depression, 89
self-actualization, 20, 22
self-amputation, 52
self-harm (non-suicidal self-injury, NSSI),
   51–57
   annual cost data, 36
   borderline personality disorder and, 135
   bulimia nervosa and, 134
   burn injuries, 52, 53–54
   comparison to suicidal behavior, 52
   cutting injuries, 52, 53
   defined, 52, 57
   deliberate foreign body ingestion,
     insertion, 54
   depression and, 86
   disposition planning, 55–56
   firearms access and, 42
   genital self-mutilation, 52
   ingestion of caustic, pharmacologic
     substances, 54–55
   interviewing a patient with, 52–53
   major self-mutilation, 55
   mental status evaluation for, 36–37

   referral for outpatient follow-up, 57
   repeat patterns, 42
   safety planning, 56
   screening tools, 86
   suicidal ideation and, 56–57
   thoughts about, 85
   triggers/warning signs, 56
   types of, 52
serotonin-norepinephrine reuptake
   inhibitors (SNRIs), 9
sexual abuse, 6, 48*f*, 120
Sheehan Suicidality Tracking Scale (S-STS),
   38
Short Blessed Test (SBT), 111
shoulder dislocation, 60
shouting, 18, 65
SIGECAPS mnemonic (*S*leep, *I*nterest,
   *G*uilt, *E*nergy, *C*oncentration,
   *A*ppetite, *P*sychomotor function,
   and *S*uicide)
single photon emission computed
   tomography (SPECT) studies, 80
Skype, 198
sleep issues, 187
   depression and, 7
   homelessness and, 8
   mania and, 7
   self-harm and, 86–87
   substance use disorders and, 76
   suicidal ideation and, 187
Social Security Disability Insurance
   Programs (SSDI), 161
social withdrawal, 80
social workers
   help navigating insurance coverages, 190
   help with homeless people, 163
   help with malingering for food, shelter, 8
   help with patients with mental illness, 158
   outpatient planning help, 191
   positive attitudes toward patients, 104
   referrals made by, 77, 162
somatic symptom disorders (SSD),
   146–148